You Can ACHIEVE NORMAL BLOOD SUGAR

DENNIS POLLOCK

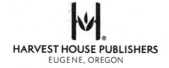

HARVEST HOUSE PUBLISHERS
EUGENE, OREGON

Cover by Bryce Williamson

Cover photo © AlexeyBlogoodf / Getty Images

You Can Achieve Normal Blood Sugar
Copyright © 2019 by Dennis Pollock
Published by Harvest House Publishers
Eugene, Oregon 97408
www.harvesthousepublishers.com

ISBN 978-0-7369-7597-1 (pbk.)
ISBN 978-0-7369-7598-8 (eBook)

Library of Congress Cataloging-in-Publication Data

Names: Pollock, Dennis, author.
Title: You can achieve normal blood sugar / Dennis Pollock.
Description: Eugene, Oregon : Harvest House Publishers, [2019]
Identifiers: LCCN 2018049667 (print) | LCCN 2018052052 (ebook) | ISBN
  9780736975988 (ebook) | ISBN 9780736975971 (paperback)
Subjects: LCSH: Diabetes--Popular works. | Diabetes--Treatment--Popular
  works. | BISAC: HEALTH & FITNESS / Healthy Living.
Classification: LCC RC660.4 (ebook) | LCC RC660.4 .P657 2019 (print) | DDC
  616.4/62--dc23
LC record available at https://lccn.loc.gov/2018049667

19 20 21 22 23 24 25 26 27 / BP-SK / 10 9 8 7 6 5 4 3 2 1

To Benedicta,
my partner in ministry and my partner in life.

Contents

Introduction

Before we get into the meat of this book, I need to give you both a spoiler and a warning. The spoiler is this: If you are serious about getting your blood sugar under control, you are almost certainly going to need to reduce your carbohydrate intake. As you read through the book and consider the many blood sugar tests I will be sharing with you, I don't think you'll have any doubt about this.

The warning is this: *If you do change your diet and you are on medication for diabetes or taking insulin, you're going to need to carefully monitor your blood sugar levels and work with a good diabetes doctor. Making major changes in your diet, especially in the carbohydrates you eat daily, will very likely require you to alter the dosage of your medication or the insulin you're taking. In most cases you will have to reduce your dosages, but your doctor will help you decide this.*

The good news is that many with type 2 diabetes may be able to eventually do away with their medication altogether. But you need to do this under the care of a doctor. I am not a doctor, and I have no business telling you what to do, what to eat, or how much medication to take. I can and will share with you what has worked for me and enabled me to steer clear of the diabetes that came rushing at me like a freight train many years ago. Whether you employ some of my own ideas and principles should be between you and your doctor. One thing I do believe this book and my story can do for you is give you new hope and motivation. Diabetes is not unbeatable! It may be a monster, but with nearly all type 2 diabetics, it is a monster with a chink in its armor. Many of us who have known its ferocity have beaten it. No, we cannot go back to eating huge bowls of ice cream and guzzling down super-sized sodas, but as long as we behave ourselves, diabetes must forever lurk in the shadows, like some rabid wolf, fearful of the bonfire that we have created for our own protection.

Read through this book. Talk to your doctor about it. Begin the process of finding your own path to healing and deliverance. And pray for God's wisdom.

My Story

I should be a full-scale, flaming, raging diabetic by now. And I would be if it were not for certain interventions I employed as I searched desperately to find answers to the terrible disease that devoured my mother's health and quality of life in her last years, and eventually shortened her life. Three major factors led me out of the morass of runaway blood sugar and into the place I am today—a place of relatively normal blood sugar and freedom from those symptoms and complications that diabetics routinely suffer. Those three factors are: 1) prayer and God's grace, 2) reading and research, and 3) an obsession to test my blood sugar after eating various meals and foods to determine precisely which foods were safe, which were "iffy," and which were dangerous for me.

My experience is personal to me, of course. It isn't my place to tell you which direction you must go in your quest to quell the raging fires of diabetes in your body. But I can share my experiences and the answers I found in the hope that, at the very least, you can be inspired that there are answers and solutions to diabetes. If you find some things that might help you in the pages of this book, share them with your diabetes doctor, and ask if any of them could work for you. I receive emails from people asking me to tell them what changes they should make in their lifestyles and diet, and I never give specific advice. Again, I am not a doctor, and I am not going to tell anyone to treat themselves. But one thing I know: I was headed for full-scale diabetes, and now I am not. I have staved off diabetes for the last 17 years, and at this point it looks as though I will live out my life without ever crossing the demarcation line that separates nondiabetics from diabetics. I am grateful.

I have written two previous books about blood sugar. The first one, *Overcoming Runaway Blood Sugar*, was an overview of what I discovered and the answers I found that enabled me to get my blood sugar back down into the normal range. The second book, *60 Ways to Lower Your Blood Sugar*, was primarily a collection of some of the dietary tips and tricks I have learned along the way as I have battled to keep my blood sugar low. After writing the second book, I was sure I had said all there was for me to say. But over time I realized that, despite all the diabetes books available, there was one approach I almost never saw. This had to do with demonstrating the effects of various foods, particularly carbohydrates, on blood sugar. Plenty of people have written about this, but almost nobody has written an entire book, loaded with overwhelming evidence through scores of blood sugar tests, that showed conclusively and irrefutably the simple truth that carbohydrates raise blood sugar like nothing else.

It has long been apparent to me that the greatest need for most diabetics and prediabetics is not so much knowledge—there is a mountain of knowledge about diabetes available today and it is constantly growing. The diabetic's ultimate need is motivation—he or she must somehow find the "want-to" to make the necessary sacrifices, substitutions, modifications, and lifestyle changes that will keep runaway blood sugar at bay and result in a long, healthy, and complication-free life. I believe that this book can be useful in supplying that motivation. We must have more than mere diabetic "sermons" preached to us; we must see with our eyes and really get the fact that our blood sugar is essentially in our hands. We can change our ways and drive blood sugars down, or we can stay on the same reckless, unhealthy, intemperate, uninformed path that has brought us to the precipice of diabetic disaster. As we read of test after test that confirm and reconfirm the folly of high-refined-carb, high-sugar living, and the efficacy of a low-carb lifestyle, we will hopefully begin to find the resolve to make the necessary changes and watch our blood sugars transformed from erratic and out of control to reasonable and very close to normal. And that is a wonderful thing.

Why I Am the Perfect Test Subject

Most of the tests you will read about in this book involve me. I have included a number of results from guest "guinea pigs," but I primarily conducted the tests on myself. The reasons for this are several. First, I was always available. No need to ask permission. Second, unlike many diabetics who have seen the light and slashed their diet to match their condition, I am not afraid to occasionally eat foods that I know will drive my blood sugar wild. I don't like to do it, and I never do this for the pleasure of eating, but for the purpose of writing this book I have eaten foods I never would have eaten otherwise—not in a thousand years.

But the most important reason I am such an ideal test subject is that I have a significant degree of insulin resistance, although my pancreas seems to work just fine. If I eat a food or a meal that I shouldn't, my blood sugar test will reflect it. If I were using young, healthy, normal subjects, they might eat a sugary food or drink a large soda, and still come out with good numbers an hour later. This doesn't really prove much, except that they are blessed with a pancreas that works beautifully and they have zero insulin resistance. And while that is very good news for them, it is not the slightest bit instructive for those of us who are diabetic or prediabetic.

I saw a YouTube video where someone stuffed himself with fruit and then tested himself at the time when his blood sugar should peak. His blood sugar score was excellent—something like 120—which led him to conclude that fruit is no problem when it comes to raising blood sugar levels. But it proved no such thing. Just because he could engorge himself with fruit and still have good numbers doesn't mean that this applies to everyone. This would be like an Olympic swimmer jumping off a ship five miles from land and then easily swimming to shore. He makes a YouTube video about his experience and declares there is no danger to being in a similar situation. He tells us that if we ever fall off a cruise ship several miles from shore, we can just do as he did. That may work beautifully for the swimmer, but for most of us, being out in the ocean miles from shore would be a death sentence. What works for the goose may not always work for the gander.

Chances are, if you are reading this book, you are either fully diabetic or at the least have significant insulin resistance, which normally leads to diabetes. *I am one of you!* In taking these tests, I represent diabetics and prediabetics everywhere who cannot eat the way other folks eat and expect to keep their blood sugar in check. When you read my scores and see my response to sugars, starches, and carbs, you will probably get a pretty accurate glimpse of how your body may respond. The good news is that in spending a few hours reading this book, you will gain insight into what has taken me many years and many hundreds (probably thousands) of blood sugar tests to discover. My admittedly biased opinion is that you cannot help but gain knowledge through walking with me and my guests as we use a simple blood sugar monitor to give us vitally important information about how our bodies process foods, and which foods serve as gasoline to the flaming torch of diabetes.

A Simple Example:
When You Can Increase Your Carbs

Let me give you an example of how I have learned to judge whether a particular meal is acceptable and safe for me. For a long time after I got the point that the major culprit that drives high blood sugar is carbohydrates, I gave up on beans. Even though they have more protein than many plant-based foods, they are still relatively high in carbs. But as I did some research I realized that beans have a pretty significant amount of fiber. One day I went through the bean section of a grocery store and checked the nutrition information on every single bag of dry beans on the shelves. I found two things. First, most beans have about the same amount of carbs per ¼ cup. There is not much difference. Second, beans have widely varying amounts of fiber. Some have far more fiber than others. Knowing that fiber was my friend, I decided to try a couple of the beans that were highest in fiber: small red beans and lentils. I had my wife, Benedicta, make a soup with them, and sure enough, using these high-fiber beans I found I could enjoy a small to medium bowl of bean soup and still keep my blood sugar at reasonable levels.

Beans reentered my life. But knowing that I would be taxing my blood sugar more than with really low-carb foods, I was a little nervous about what I could have with them. Somehow a bowl of beans seemed incomplete by itself. I knew that some version of low-carb bread would probably work. A stick of celery with peanut butter seemed to have little effect on my blood sugar, so that would probably be okay too. But what about an apple with peanut butter? A full-sized, entire apple was out of the question, having around 25 grams of carbs. But what about half an apple with some peanut butter on it?

On two successive days I did two tests on myself to see the effect of beans plus these two additional foods: one celery stick with peanut butter and one half of an apple with peanut butter. I normally test my blood sugar one hour after my last bite of food. In this case I waited an hour and 15 minutes (beans take slightly longer to peak your blood sugar, thus the longer wait time), and tested again. To my great delight, both of these foods proved okay for me.

With the lentil soup plus celery and peanut butter, my blood sugar peaked at 112. No problems there. And with the lentil soup plus apple with peanut butter (I ended up eating three-fourths of the apple because it was a very small apple), my blood sugar peaked at 119. That was exciting! I now had evidence that here were two meals I could eat for lunch or dinner that would not offend my pancreas or cause my blood sugar levels to rise so high they would be doing serious damage to my organs.

LENTIL SOUP TEST		
	Soup Plus Celery with Peanut Butter	Soup Plus ¾ Apple with Peanut Butter
Before Eating	94	96
After 1 Hour	112	119
Total Blood Sugar Rise	18 mg/dl	23 mg/dl

Summary: I do not have to give up on beans! What a blessing it is to know that moderately high-carb beans are back on the menu, although in moderate portions. Even with three-fourths of a small apple, my blood sugar behaved itself. Now I had a couple of lunches I could enjoy guilt-free in the future!

What I'm talking about here are two key factors that empower us to overcome runaway blood sugar: *knowledge* and *motivation*. After tests like these, I receive knowledge I did not have before. By continually testing myself an hour or an hour and a half after eating, I learn what is safe and what is dangerous, what I can and should be eating, and what I cannot and should not ever touch. In this case I added two meals to my "repertoire" of recipes that I can pull out at any time and enjoy without guilt and without harm. Of course, no one wants to live on bean soup and celery or apples with peanut butter. But this is just one example. When you do this again and again, you begin to collect meals and categorize them in your mind. One test is probably not enough, so I would test myself several times to make sure. If after several times your numbers are good, you can be pretty sure that these meals make up a part of your "approved" list.

And seeing those numbers provides incredible motivation as well as information. High numbers make me sick! I hate them! And when I see certain foods giving me consistently high, unsafe numbers, I instinctively avoid those foods or meals. I know that if I eat them, the story will have a sad ending. How different this is from those who never test themselves, or only test themselves occasionally in the mornings. They have no information, no motivation, and no clue as to what is going on in their bodies. And so they continue in the same, miserable dietary habits that got them into the mess in the first place.

How I Entered the World of Runaway Blood Sugar

Although I didn't know it at the time, I began experiencing symptoms of blood sugar problems while I was in my early thirties. One of the first signs that I was headed for trouble was a jittery, nervous, uneasy feeling I would get near noon after eating a big pancake breakfast. The pancakes were swimming in a sugary syrup, and I was probably loading my system with nearly 100 grams of carbs, but in those days I knew nothing of such things. All I knew was that when I had those big pancake breakfasts I would usually feel funny a few hours afterward. Often, I would get shaky to the point that my handwriting, never very good, would deteriorate. I didn't think about diabetes; I just assumed it was "one of those things."

Within a few years I started to have episodes when I felt lightheaded and close to passing out. It was always in connection with eating sugary, high-carb meals. Once I ate a personal-sized packaged fruit pie, which I now know is one of the highest carb snacks you can eat—around 60 grams of carbs. Don't ask me why, but after eating the fruit pie I then ate about half of a giant-sized chocolate bar. Shortly after that, while sitting at my desk, my head began to spin. I felt as though I was about to faint. The feeling passed in a couple of minutes, but it was scary and made me wonder what in the world was going on.

In my late thirties through my forties, these experiences increased. It was never an everyday thing, but it was often enough to really bother me. Once, after eating a lot of pizza and washing it down with Coke, I went with my family to our local Walmart. While walking through the store, I had a strong feeling that I was losing it, that I would soon pass out. I immediately left the store and sat in my car while my family shopped. It was unnerving.

I responded to these scares by increasing my exercising and cutting back on sugary sweets. It bought me a few years and I felt better. But by my late forties the episodes began coming back and getting worse. What really grabbed my attention was an incident at church. That morning I had eaten a large bowl of raisin bran–type cereal (which most people would assume to be a healthy cereal but is in fact loaded with carbs). Just before church was over I got out of my seat, intending to go by the church bookstore before I left. As I walked I suddenly felt terribly weak and faint. I headed for the bathroom, thinking I could recover in there. I never quite made it to the bathroom. As I got close, knowing I about to pass out, I put my back up against the wall and slid down to the floor. This time I really did pass out. I awoke with a nurse cradling my head, and paramedics soon arrived. They tested my blood sugar, and it was so low it didn't give a numerical score. It simply read "LO," which means you are dangerously low—to the point where death is possible. They gave me some snacks and fruit juice and stayed with me until it rose into the 70s. They urged me to go to the hospital, but I was too cheap for that, and instead went home and went to bed. After a nap I felt normal again.

Raisin Bran—Not as Healthy as You Might Think

Let's pause and talk about raisin bran–type cereals. If you bother to look at the nutritional information on Kellogg's Raisin Bran, you will find something like 46 grams of carbs for 1 cup of cereal. Granted, 7 grams are fiber grams, which may be deducted from your "net gram" carb count, but that still leaves 39 grams of carbs for 1 cup of cereal. That's already too much, and then there's the problem that hardly anybody would eat 1 cup of cereal for breakfast. Have you ever measured out 1 cup of cereal and then poured that amount into your bowl? You will have the scrawniest, saddest, most pathetic bowl of cereal imaginable! When I had that large bowl of cereal, I probably ate more than 2 cups. When you add an additional 12 grams of carbs for the milk, I was probably ingesting around 100 grams of carbs that morning in that one "healthy" bowl of cereal. That is more carbs than you would get by eating three regular-sized *Snicker* bars! Thinking I was doing myself a favor by eating a bran cereal, I was in fact challenging my poor, overworked pancreas terribly. And fainting at church was the result.

The Cereal That Nearly Killed Me!

Recently, I tested myself with the same cereal that sent my blood sugar so low it nearly killed me. Pouring the cereal into the bowl, I couldn't help but notice just how "healthy" it looks. The dark-brown color and rough texture of the bran flakes make you feel that you are one with nature as you eat this food. And the raisins are surely an added bonus: you are getting the nutrients of fruit along with the roughage of the bran. It just looks like a wonderfully, crunchy, healthy breakfast. I filled my bowl with cereal using a 1-cup measure. In my large bowl I was able to put a little over 2 cups of cereal and still the bowl wasn't full. Nevertheless, I knew I would be taxing my pancreas in a big way. Those 2-plus cups of cereal, along with the regular milk I poured over it, represented nearly 100 grams of carbohydrates.

I was eating this cereal for the first time in 17 years. Apart from doing the research for this book, I normally would never eat this cereal, and I will probably never touch it again for the rest of my life. But for this one experiment, I would break my own rules. Strange, isn't it, that what I was doing in eating a bowl of cereal would not appear the least bit risky or foolish in probably 99 percent of people's eyes, but for me, I was really going out on a limb. My pre-meal, fasting blood sugar registered 100, a decent number for me. I knew that after eating this meal, my blood sugar would rise significantly. I have tested myself enough to know about how many carbs I can handle at one setting, and 100 grams was way over my limit.

I was eating the same exact breakfast that had nearly killed me. I could not say that I enjoyed the cereal. It tasted great, but the pleasure of the meal was muted by the knowledge that I was ingesting a food that would push my pancreas to the limits and raise my blood sugar far beyond my target boundary of 140. An hour after finishing my breakfast, I tested myself with my trusty blood sugar monitor. I didn't have to wait long to see the results. Within seconds the monitor read 196—surely a sickening number and one that no one would ever want to see show up on their monitor. *My blood sugar had risen a whopping 96 points in a little over an hour!*

Checking my blood sugar a few hours later, I saw it was starting to dip low. It read 73, which is not dangerous, but that is an unnatural level for me, and it was impossible to tell how much lower it would go. I wasn't going to take a chance on the same thing happening as before, so I ate some cheese and a few peanuts to ease my blood sugar down gradually rather than have it come crashing down way too low. The 196 on my monitor was ugly, nasty, and depressing, but it wasn't a surprise. Whether they come from bread, candy, apple pie with ice cream, or a large hamburger with lots of French fries, 100 grams of carbs is too much. In fact, 50 grams is too much as far as I'm concerned.

A Lower-Carb Cereal

When I test myself, I love to set up contrasting tests to demonstrate the superiority of low carb over high carb. So after bombarding my body with carbs and sugar that morning, I set up another test the next morning. This time I wanted to demonstrate how I learned to eat cereal in a way that does not send my blood sugar into orbit. I have gone through the cereal departments of grocery stores looking for the lowest-carb cereal I can find. The sad truth is that there are no truly low-carb cereals to be had. There used to be one or two you could find about 17 years ago, when low-carb was more fashionable than it is today. The closest I could come to a low-carb cereal was Special K High Protein cereal and the various versions of Cheerios-type cereals (Cheerios itself and the generic versions).

Both of these cereals have around 20 grams of carbs per cup, which is really not low-carb but was the best I could find. Granted, I could order some genuinely low-carb cereals from low-carb internet websites, but they are far costlier, and by the time you include the shipping you are paying perhaps three times the price of grocery store cereal.

The way I keep my cereal from raising my blood sugar through the roof is threefold. First, I eat less of it. These days I use a small bowl and don't even fill that to the top. Second, as mentioned, I eat the lowest-carb cereals I can find. And third, I make my own milk, using about one-fourth part heavy whipping cream and three-fourths part water. This means cutting my milk carbs from around 12 to perhaps 3. (One key to victory over high blood sugar is to save on carbs every way you possibly can. Every carb you can avoid, do it!).

You may be thinking, *You're not getting too much cereal!* And the answer is no, I'm not. You can't. Cereal is made from grains. There is no cereal made from steak or eggs, or cucumbers. Cereal is all grain, and it is nearly all carbs. There is just no way you can pig out on cereal if you hope to keep your blood sugar under control. Of course, you don't want to leave the table nearly as hungry as you were before eating, so when I have my small bowl of cereal, I always eat a few peanuts. These help to fill me up, and still I get to enjoy the sweet flavor from the cereal. The fat in the nuts also helps reduce the blood sugar spike. You may say, "Why don't you just give up on cereal altogether?" That wouldn't be a bad idea, and many diabetics do just that, but I have loved cereal all my life, and it would be painful to think I could never have the taste of cereal the rest of my days. Besides, it makes for a nice, quick breakfast when I'm in a hurry.

So I ate my small bowl of Toasted Oats (a generic version of Cheerios), had a handful of peanuts, and drank my coffee. Before the meal my fasting blood sugar read 102. One hour after the meal it registered 128. I was satisfied. I had eaten one of my favorite foods in a manner that kept my blood sugar within my prescribed boundaries, and all was well. Life is good!

HIGH-CARB VS. LOWER-CARB CEREAL TEST (WITH MILK)		
	Raisin Bran (Large Bowl)	Toasted Oats (Small Bowl) with Handful of Peanuts
Before Eating	100	102
After 1 Hour	196	128
Total Blood sugar Rise	96 mg/dl	26 mg/dl

Summary: With its emphasis on raisins and bran, one might think that raisin bran would be a great food. But for diabetics it just ain't so. Seventeen years after it nearly drove my blood sugar crazy, it's still a serious problem for me. Despite appearances, high carb is high carb! My blood sugar results for the Toasted Oats demonstrate that when it comes to carbs, less is more!

Since the time I did this experiment and wrote about it, I have found a wonderful substitute for regular breakfast cereal. In fact, it's so good that I have pretty much given up on cereal altogether. It involves the lowly chia seed. I take a traditional "chia seed pudding" (type that in the YouTube search box, and you'll find numerous recipes) and then add several different kinds of nuts to it along with a few blueberries and some Stevia. It's good—so good that it has finally given me the will-power to give up on regular cereal.

Getting Worse and Getting Desperate

My blood sugar episodes became more and more frequent. It became obvious that something was seriously wrong with me and that I desperately needed some answers. I happened to run across an article by a man who claimed he had a total cure for diabetes. His "cure" was not at all complicated—just go vegetarian and stay away from meat altogether. He sounded like he knew what he was talking about, so I immediately dropped meat from my diet and went vegetarian. It sounds impulsive to change my diet so radically simply on the basis of a few claims of success, but I was desperate.

No more hamburgers, no more chicken, no more bacon. It was a radical change, but what I didn't realize was that when most people become vegetarians, they substitute carbs for meat, which is exactly what I did. And, not surprisingly, my high and low blood sugar episodes increased exponentially. One evening when we had relatives over, my brother-in-law bought fried chicken for everyone. Trying to be a good boy, I passed on the chicken and made myself some spaghetti with a meatless sauce. Within a couple of hours, the shaking and all those strange unnerving feelings began. It was worse than usual this time, and I tested my blood sugar to see what was happening. My blood sugar reading was around 40 mg/dl. I knew this was dangerously low, so I chugged a soda immediately. I waited a little while and then tested myself again. This time the monitor read in the 170s. I lay down, but the trembling increased, and while the family enjoyed a movie in the living room, I was in my bed shaking like a leaf and wondering what in the world was wrong with me.

Another terrifying experience happened while I was at work. I don't remember what I had eaten for breakfast that morning, but it must have been loaded with carbs because a few hours later, just before lunchtime, it started happening again. By now I knew the signs and the way my body felt when the bottom dropped out of my blood sugar. The last thing I wanted was to faint at work, so with my office door closed I grabbed a bag of chips I kept around for just such emergencies. In my desperation to get my blood sugar up fast, I stuffed as many chips into my mouth as I could. The problem was, while I was in the process of chewing the huge mouthful of chips, one of my coworkers knocked at my door, telling me it was time for lunch. He often did this, and I always replied to his knock by saying, "I'm coming."

But this time I couldn't say anything—my mouth was still stuffed with the chips, and I could not get them down very quickly. My friend waited patiently to hear my reply, but it took me what seemed like forever to finally chew up the chips and utter a garbled, "Okay, I'll be there in a minute." It would have been funny if it wasn't so scary.

Once I had to go home before lunch just to sleep off my trembling and shaking. After a while I began eating something every few hours to stave off the symptoms of crashing blood sugar. It was a miserable existence, never knowing when I might be near fainting and not really knowing what to do about it. A combination of a high-sugar and high-carb diet was making my blood sugar bounce up and down like a yo-yo. I now know that my problem was an overreacting pancreas and severe insulin resistance. But in those days I had little idea what was going on.

First Response

Having no health insurance, I resisted going to see a doctor for quite a while, but eventually I broke down and made an appointment with a doctor I picked at random (she was nearby and had a nice name). The problem was, she was a general practitioner and not a diabetes doctor—again my cheapness was shining through! As I recall, she took my fasting blood sugar, which was normal, and asked me a series of questions from a prepared list. She didn't seem to have much of an idea what was going on. However, she did give me a little good advice. Learning I was eating a vegetarian diet, she urged me to eat foods with protein when I was having a meal that was mostly carbohydrates. This I began to do, and my episodes slowed down a bit.

Almost from the beginning of these blood sugar fluctuations, even before I began to test myself, I had a sneaking suspicion that my problem might have something to do with diabetes. My mother had been diabetic in her later years, and it had taken a terrible toll on her. As with so many diabetics, she had poor circulation, especially in her legs and feet. It became painful for her to walk any distance, and even when she was at the mall with my sister, she would have to sit down and rest a while after walking through a few stores. Doctors told her that her veins were collapsing and put in stents and tried different procedures to save her legs, but to no avail. The day came when she was forced to have one leg amputated, and within a couple of years, the other leg was also amputated above the knee. This time there was an infection, and it was necessary for the doctors to cut off even more of her leg. It was a miserable time for her. After her first leg was gone, she used a prosthetic and could still walk, but after the second amputation she was confined to a wheelchair.

Mom tested her blood at times and, as far as I know, she never had super-high numbers. But the diabetes was merciless, and it spoiled the last ten years of her life. My dad, who was nine years older than her, was faithful to take her wherever she needed to go and to stay with her almost constantly, but when he died, she was forced to stay at home by herself and get along as best she could until my sister came home from work. Mostly she lay in bed. She managed to live to the age of 80, but the last decade of her life was not a very happy season for her. Thank God she is in heaven now, and her struggles are a thing of the past.

As I dealt with wildly fluctuating blood sugar, all of this was in my mind. I feared I was going down the same path as Mom, and I was starting earlier in life than she did. It was not a pleasant prospect. I really needed some answers, and I eventually found them. As I read books about blood sugar and diabetes, I found that there seemed to be two very different approaches to taming the monster. One was a meatless, low-fat diet, and the other was based on significantly reducing carbohydrates in the diet.

At this point I had no biases. I did not favor one approach over the other. I just wanted something that worked. If I had to eat sawdust for every meal and could be assured it would keep me healthy, I would have done it. It was when I began doing pre-meal and post-meal blood sugar tests that the light began to come on. Almost everybody with blood sugar problems tests themselves at times, but many people limit themselves to the standard fasting blood sugar test—the blood sugar level you get when you test in the morning after eating nothing all night. This can give you a general idea about things, but it is not that helpful for two reasons.

Problems with Testing Fasting Blood Sugar

First, testing our fasting blood sugar alone may be misleading. In my case, during all of those early days when my blood sugar was seesawing back and forth, my fasting blood sugar was in the normal range. An uninformed doctor, seeing this, might well tell me, "You are okay. Your blood sugar fluctuations are normal." But I was not at all okay. I was heading for disaster. With certain meals my blood sugar would skyrocket well out of the normal range, and then a few hours later it would drop precipitously to dangerous levels. I discovered all of this when I began to test myself frequently.

Second, even if your fasting blood sugar is quite high, you gain no information about what is making it high. What foods are driving your blood sugar up so powerfully? Is it cucumbers, or green beans, or potatoes, or chips, or avocadoes, or steak, or rice, or salad? Who knows? Thankfully, your blood sugar monitor can tell you this, if you have enough sense and enough patience to test yourself frequently and at the appropriate times.

As I researched and learned about another major school of thought that allowed for meat but strongly restricted carbs, I determined to allow my blood sugar monitor to decide for me which version of a diabetes fix I would embrace. I also read somewhere about the importance of obtaining a post-meal blood sugar reading. This involved eating a particular food or meal, waiting an hour to an hour and a half after finishing your meal, and then testing to determine your glucose level as your blood sugar peaked from the meal just eaten. It was this practice of testing my blood sugar peaks that led me out of the darkness and into the light of normal blood sugar.

Beginning of the End—and the Beginning of the Beginning!

My "aha" moment came on a trip when I tested myself after two very different meals. The first was a large hamburger (with a very large bun) along with corn chips. My post-meal number was around 185, which depressed me greatly. I remember going for a walk after I tested myself, hoping that the physical exertion would help get my blood sugar down. I was heartsick over the high number and determined to eat something at my next meal that would give me a better score (sounds sort of like a baseball game, doesn't it?).

The next meal I tested was a chef's salad. I ate almost none of the croutons. This time my post-meal score was somewhere around 118. I was euphoric! I made a change in the food I ate, and my blood sugar monitor reflected that change in a very positive way. Soon I was bursting with hope and with a very simple thought: *I can do this! I can find out which foods are safe and which drive my blood sugar crazy. And then I'll just start eating the safe foods and passing on the dangerous ones.* This was not a stroke of genius. I do not consider it at all brilliant. It was simply common sense.

It worked beautifully. Within a very short time my fluctuating blood sugar and near-fainting episodes were a thing of the past. I no longer had to eat every few hours just to keep my blood sugar from crashing. And I wasn't experiencing those terrible high numbers that spelled the coming of full-fledged diabetes. This was around 17 years ago, and I am still doing great. Although I read quite a few books on the subject, the ultimate judge, umpire, and dictator for me was my handy-dandy, friendly little neighborhood blood sugar monitor. The monitor cost around $20, and a package of strips about $20 more.

Re-Creating Earlier Glucose Tests

Below is a test I did with the help of two dear friends. This was such a contrast from those early tests when I was sick, scared, and desperately seeking answers. What a difference a little knowledge can make. We contrasted a high-carb meal with a low-carb meal. Before we even began, I was already certain of how these tests would turn out. I did not know the exact numbers we would get, but I knew one thing for sure: the high-carb meal would spike our blood sugar significantly, and the low-carb meal would not. I was not surprised.

Recreating Those First Two Enlightening Tests

Recently I invited a couple I knew, Fred and Lynda Lindstrom, to join me in re-creating these two meals that were so illuminating to me. The first meal was the one that depressed me so much: the large hamburger and large helping of corn chips. Fred has been diagnosed as prediabetic, and his wife, Lynda, is essentially normal. She sometimes tests her blood sugar in the mornings and gets readings in the high 80s and low 90s. They graciously agreed to eat the same meal that drove my blood sugar so high around 17 years ago to see what it did to their blood sugar levels.

Before we ate, we tested our blood sugar to discover our starting point. We all tested at a decent level. Lynda scored an 88 and Fred tested at 101. Mine was at 104, and just for fun we tested our cameraman, Jordan, who is in his late twenties, and he scored 82. Then we had our meal. The Whoppers were good, and I have to admit that the Fritos tasted pretty great as well. Normally I would never touch chips, but for this little experiment I made an exception. It was a big meal, and Fred had a hard time finishing it. We waited until we had all completed our meal, and then set the timer for one hour.

After an hour we began testing ourselves, starting with our cameraman. His blood sugar rose around 60 points, which left us wondering, *If this young man in his twenties can increase that much, how much will our blood sugar rise?* Lynda's blood sugar tested at 159, a 71-point rise. Fred tested at 174, a 73-point rise in about an hour. Mine was a bit of a surprise. It rose to 150, which was a lower peak than that original meal so long ago. It appears that in all these years, my body's blood sugar response is at least as efficient, if not more efficient than it was. That is exciting!

LARGE HAMBURGER AND CORN CHIPS TEST			
	Dennis	Fred	Lynda
Before Eating	104	101	88
After 1 Hour	150	174	159
Total Blood sugar Rise	46 mg/dl	73 mg/dl	71 mg/dl

Summary: There was nothing that tasted sweet in this meal. What raised our blood sugar significantly were the starches: the buns and the chips. Without candy, cake, or pie, we were still over the limits of blood sugar safety. And none of us were true diabetics!

The American Association of Clinical Endocrinologists has recommended that we keep our blood sugar from rising above 140 in order to avoid diabetic complications.[1] After the hamburger and corn chips, we had all risen above that. Now, if this type of meal was our normal way of eating—that is, if we constantly ate meals loaded with carbs, plus had high-carb snacks here and there, along with sodas, fruit juice, and other sweet drinks (the way many Americans eat and drink)—we would be at diabetic levels much of the day, doing severe damage to our bodies over the course of time.

Here's something worth considering. As I mentioned, none of us are true diabetics. Fred and I have hovered in the prediabetic range for years, and Lynda wouldn't even qualify as a prediabetic. If this meal affected us this way, what do you suppose it would do to a real diabetic, with a fasting blood sugar of, say, 140 or 150? Almost surely he or she would end up over 200 on the post-test. And keep in mind that few Americans would eat this meal the way we did. Most would have a soda with it, adding an additional 40 grams of carbs. Some would want a dessert of some kind at the end of the meal, adding more carbs still and raising their blood sugar even higher.

A Second Test with Fred and Lynda

Fred, Lynda, and I got together a few days later to do a second test. This time I chose a meal that was low in carbohydrates. We went to a pancake restaurant, not to eat pancakes, but to eat a large omelet. Before entering the restaurant, we tested our blood sugar in Fred's car. We all tested in a decent range. Our meal at the restaurant was a large omelet stuffed with beef, bacon, sausage, green peppers, onions, and cheese. After our meal, we went to Fred and Lynda's house, and when one hour had passed after our last bite of omelet, we tested ourselves. The results were a whole lot more pleasant this time.

Now, both meals were extremely filling; we walked away from the table totally stuffed both times. But that is where the similarity ended.

The contrast could hardly have been greater. Fred went up 73 points with the burger meal but dropped 21 points with the omelet. Lynda's blood sugar rose 71 points with the burger meal and dropped 4 points with the omelet. And I rose 46 points eating the burger and chips but dropped 2 points after having the omelet.

OMELET TEST			
	Dennis	Fred	Lynda
Before Eating	92	98	87
After 1 Hour	90	77	83
Total Blood sugar Rise	-2 mg/dl	-21 mg/dl	-4 mg/dl

Summary: What a contrast! In this case each one of us had our blood sugar drop by the one-hour mark. The omelet proved a kinder, gentler food for our blood sugar processing system. If ever there was evidence to choose eggs over chips, this is surely it!

Low-Carb Intervention

Could it be any plainer? The foods we eat possess three essential types of macronutrients: protein, carbohydrates, and fats. Of these three, the only one that has a major impact on blood sugar are the carbohydrates. Fats do not raise blood sugar at all. Proteins can raise blood sugar, but for most of us, it is a very slight, almost imperceptible rise. But carbohydrates are an entirely different matter. Raising blood sugar is what they do; it is their specialty, their unique domain. And for people with diabetes or prediabetes, the more carbs you eat, the higher your blood sugar will soar (especially when those carbs are refined and processed). It comes down to a very simple formula: Eat a small amount of carbs, get a small blood sugar rise. Eat a medium amount of carbs, get a bigger blood sugar rise. Eat a meal with a large amount of carbs, get a whopping rise in blood sugar. And, sadly, we must also add: Build a lifestyle on eating refined, processed carbs, carbs, and more carbs, and you will have an excellent chance of becoming diabetic and destroying your health, spoiling your latter days, and shortening your life.

But when carbs are restricted, blood sugars will drop. Dr. Sarah

Hallberg, medical director of Virta Health (a successful diabetes center) says in her YouTube lecture, which has garnered millions of views: "Low-carb intervention works so fast that we can literally pull people off hundreds of units of insulin in days to weeks."[2]

And while I'm quoting doctors, let me give you one more quote that, while very simple, was incredibly powerful in getting my attention when I was first looking for answers to runaway blood sugar. It is by the late Dr. Robert Atkins, who wrote, "Your blood-glucose level doesn't sharply rise and fall when you sit down to eat a Cobb salad. But it does just that when you chow down a slice of pie."[3]

Now, that's not profound, it's not deep, it's not rocket science…but it is unquestionably, indisputably, and incontrovertibly true. But we don't have to stop there. We could insert all kinds of substitutions into that equation. Your blood sugar won't sharply rise and fall when you eat an avocado, but it will when you eat a doughnut. It won't rise and fall when you eat eggs and ham, but it will when you gobble up a bunch of pancakes drenched in syrup. And on and on we could go.

Our Desperate Need for Hope

Do you remember when you were a kid and you had the misfortune to be on a softball team that was totally mismatched against a much better team? At first you probably didn't realize just how mismatched you were. Maybe after the first inning the score was 6 to 1, and you thought, *Well, we didn't do so great this inning, but we'll get it back next inning.* But after the second inning, the score was something like 15 to 2. You realized that you couldn't possibly win the game. You were beaten from the beginning. But you still had five more innings to play. What did you do? Chances are, you got sloppy. You didn't try too hard, you goofed around, you got kind of silly. You stopped taking the game seriously, because in your mind you were already a loser.

This is precisely the way many people feel about their lives, and this is how some people feel about this area of blood sugar. They assume they are just unlucky. They have the misfortune to be a diabetic, or they know they soon will be, and they sadly resign themselves to their fate. They make a few token efforts, but they never really do too much, because in their mind they are already a loser. They have lost hope.

The purpose of this book is to say, in as many ways as I can say it and using many different blood sugar tests, you don't have to be a loser. There is hope for you! And hope is such a beautiful thing. As horrible as diabetes is, there is one really good thing about the type 2 variety. It normally responds quickly and beautifully to the right kinds of behaviors and lifestyle changes. With cancer and emphysema and so many other diseases, all you can do is go to the doctor and hope you are one of the lucky ones who beats the odds. But with type 2 diabetes, or if you are prediabetic, the actions you take and the foods you eat (and refuse to eat) can make a huge difference, and they can determine whether this disease destroys your life, or you end up living a long and healthy life. And just knowing this can turn your tepid, sluggish, listless attempts at overcoming your condition into a raging inferno of motivation and determination that will drastically change and enhance your prospects. Victory tastes a whole lot sweeter than failure, and once you taste some victory in this area of blood sugar, it will be almost impossible to stop you.

2

Let's Talk About
Blood Sugar Testing

In the previous chapter we looked at some of my own history with runaway blood sugar and how I found answers that have helped me keep diabetes at bay for all these years since then. In this chapter we are going to be talking a little more specifically about the actual process of blood sugar testing: the why, the how, and the when.

But before we get into the nature of testing today, let's take a look at how the glucose monitor developed. We have known about diabetes for a long time, but it wasn't until the 1800s that researchers figured out that this disease correlates to excess sugar in the blood and then passes out of the body through urine. Once this was understood, physicians and researchers found crude ways to measure sugar in the urine, which would be a dead giveaway that the individual had diabetes. In time, strips were developed that would be dipped in urine and would turn black if excess sugar was present. This was helpful for diagnostic purposes but didn't provide assistance in bringing about an improvement for the diabetic. Nor was it precise. In those days there were two essential test results: the strip turns black, meaning you have a lot of sugar in your urine, or the strip does not, meaning you don't have too much. There was no talk about prediabetics in those days.

As time marched on, and we passed the midpoint of the twentieth century, there was a new, exciting breakthrough. A division of Miles Laboratories (known mostly in those days for producing Alka Seltzer and One-a-Day vitamins) began experimenting with the creation of a glucose monitor that would measure, not one's urine, but one's blood. By the mid-sixties they had produced a reasonably accurate monitor. It was a heavy device, weighing around three pounds, and it was marketed to doctors and hospitals. There was little thought that it would be used by private individuals. However, they were willing to sell it to type 1 diabetics if they had a prescription from their doctor.

Diabetes, Meet Mr. Bernstein

The realm of diabetic knowledge took a quantum leap forward when a skinny little engineer saw an advertisement for the monitor in a medical magazine. He was a type 1 diabetic, and his diabetes was killing him. He was experiencing all sorts of diabetic complications. He often passed out from hypoglycemic episodes. He had severe burning in his chest after every meal, and frequently all day long. He would consume around 200 Rolaid tablets per week in an effort to control the burning. His eyes became so bad that if he wanted to go to the movies, he had to sit in a back row for about half an hour, until his eyes became adjusted to the darkness, at which point he could go down farther into the theater. Even though he wasn't even middle aged, his heart was already showing signs of failure. He was a mess, and he was desperate.

At that time the Ames glucose monitor was being marketed to hospital emergency rooms. It was a way for doctors to assess unconscious patients and determine whether they were drunk or in a diabetic coma. This new device could tell them in one minute, through sticking a finger and getting a drop of blood, the glucose level in the blood. When Bernstein read of the new device, he was fascinated. Until then he had not been able to control his blood sugar from wild fluctuations, but this glucose monitor could be invaluable in helping him figure out what was going on with his body and how he could avoid such extreme highs and lows in blood sugar. Bernstein's wife was a physician, and so, with her permission, he used her official stationery to order the blood sugar monitor at a cost of $650. (This was in 1969. That same amount would be $4,500 today.)

When the device arrived, Bernstein went to work and began measuring his blood glucose levels many times throughout the day. Having a brilliant and inquisitive mind, he conducted tests on himself to determine such things as: 1) How much would one unit of insulin lower his blood sugar? And 2) how much would one gram of carbohydrate raise his blood sugar? Being a type 1 diabetic with virtually no insulin secretion from his pancreas, he was able to determine very precise numbers to these and other questions.

As he tested the causes of his blood sugar rise, he found that his biggest increase was after lunch, which was his highest carbohydrate meal. A simple idea resulted, an insight that has enabled him to live to be an old man and stay healthy from that point to the present. His idea was this: the only possible way to precisely control his blood sugar was to significantly limit his carbohydrates and make the small number of carbs he was eating match perfectly with the insulin he gave himself. He found that when he ate high-carb meals or ate meals with even moderate amounts of carbs (which quickly converted to sugar, such as bread), there was no possible way to keep his blood sugar in check, even by taking insulin before the meal. He learned that to get precise blood sugar control he would have to (a) ingest a very small amount of carbohydrates, and (b) only eat foods with carbs that did not quickly break down. In other words, vegetable carbs were okay (but not potatoes or corn); bread carbs, fruit carbs, and sugar carbs were not.

Mystery Solved

After much trial and error, and innumerable blood sugar tests, Bernstein found a system that worked beautifully. The hypoglycemic episodes and passing out came to an end. Most of his diabetic complications completely reversed themselves. He gained weight and felt great. By measuring the very few carbs in his meals and the insulin units he took to deal with those carbs, he not only knew what his blood sugar was throughout the day, but he gained the ability to essentially make it what he wanted it to be. And what he wanted it to be was normal.

Bernstein was euphoric. He had discovered a solution that no doctor in those days seemed to be even considering. With all the zeal of a new convert, he went around trying to talk to doctors and get articles published in medical journals. No one would listen to him. First, he was not a doctor; he was an engineer. Second, he was advocating a method that seemed novel and strange. And third, since the average person in those days had neither the money nor the opportunity to own a glucose monitor, it seemed highly impractical. When he tried to publish an article detailing his method for controlling blood sugar in the *Journal of the American Medical Association*, they rejected it, telling him, "No one in his right mind would let an electrical device tell him how to treat his diabetes."[1] Another medical journal rejected him, telling him that there was no evidence that there was any value to normalizing blood sugar.

Bernstein was a man who clung to his new discovery like a pit bull. Since the medical folks wanted nothing to do with him, he decided, "If you can't beat them, join them." He went to medical school and earned an MD. He became a doctor, specializing in diabetes. Now when he spoke, at least some people listened to him. And he had not only a great theory and lots of facts at his disposal; he had his own powerful testimony. And he has devoted his life to speaking—no, make that shouting—to the diabetics in the world for many years now, declaring that there is hope for all.

Since those days there has been a quantum leap in the evolution of the blood sugar monitors. Today they are smaller, lighter, and cheaper than ever before. They require less blood and are more accurate. In short, there is no valid reason for diabetics and prediabetics not to test themselves. The feedback and information these tests provide are so valuable it would be incredibly foolish not to test.

My Own Case

I can powerfully identify with Richard Bernstein, although in many ways we could not be more different. He is a type 1 diabetic, and I have kept myself in the prediabetic range for 17 years at this point. He became a doctor, while I have no desire to become a doctor. He watches his carbs with perfect precision, allowing himself 6 grams of carbs for breakfast, 12 for lunch, and 12 for dinner. He is so exact that he often will repeat the same meals for weeks and months until he gets tired of them, just because he knows the exact amount of insulin to take with that meal. He is fanatical in determining exactly how many carbs each meal gives him, and 12 is his absolute limit.

I am not nearly so strict with myself. But, as I said, I do identify with Dr. Bernstein and consider him a true "hero" in the realm of diabetes. He is doing what works for him and has helped great numbers of diabetics get into the normal range. The main reason I identify with him is that I also worked my way down from runaway blood sugar largely as a result of testing myself and discovering which foods cause the highest blood sugar peaks. I don't take insulin and never have. But I know that I could easily be diabetic if I ate the way normal Americans eat.

The one thing that led me out of the darkness of wildly fluctuating blood sugar is the concept of post-meal testing. I still don't remember exactly how I came across the idea. But wherever the idea came from, it was a lifesaver for me.

Simple but Effective

When I started testing my blood sugar after meals and particular foods, the blinders came off and I began to see what foods were doing, or not doing, to me. Even though I was having terrible blood sugar episodes, my blood sugar levels were decent. My fasting blood sugar was normal. This didn't really tell me anything, except that I had not yet reached the point where I was fully diabetic (getting several fasting blood sugar scores of 126 mg/dl is considered the mark of a true diabetic, although most doctors look more at the A1C score these days, 6.5 or higher on two separate occasions means diabetes). The A1C test provides an average of the glucose levels in your blood over the last three months. In my case neither my fasting blood sugar nor my A1C scores have ever shown me to be a full-fledged diabetic, thank the Lord!

But although I may not have been officially classified as a diabetic, I was surely having serious blood sugar issues and showing definite indications of insulin resistance. And as I began to test my post-meal blood sugar peaks, it didn't take long to figure some things out. Of course, what I was learning was something any non-biased diabetes doctor could have told me, which was that starches and sugars (essentially carbohydrates, and especially refined, processed carbs) raised blood sugar, while low-carb foods and meals did not raise it very much. This was no brilliant discovery, but for me it was life-saving and tremendously encouraging. Eat one type of meal and watch my blood sugar levels approach 200. Eat another meal, and this time my blood sugar levels don't even top 120.

Testing my blood sugar became very natural for me. I did it in my home, I did it in my car, and I did it wherever I needed to do it, once my alarm or watch told me that an hour had passed since I'd finished that last bite. And as I ate and tested and ate and tested, my diet began to change. I loved those low numbers and hated the high ones. Every 180, 190, or 200 made me sick and made me determined never to eat that meal again. And every 105, 115, or 125 thrilled me and gave me a powerful desire to eat that meal again and again and again.

I didn't use expensive blood sugar monitors; I couldn't afford to. In those days I used cheap little units I bought at a local grocery store. They may not have been as accurate as some of the higher-priced models, but they gave me a good idea when I was inbounds and when I had strayed far out of bounds. Under God, I owe my life, my eyes, my kidneys, and my legs to those cheap little monitors of those early days.

Fundamentals of Glucose Monitoring

Let's consider the main components and aspects of testing for blood sugar levels. There are three factors today that make blood sugar tests superior now than at any time in the past. First, the testing equipment is readily available, something that has only been true in the last generation. For thousands of years there was no way to monitor your blood sugar. Today there is.

Second, it is cheap. The monitors themselves are sold for very little. What these companies hope is that you will stay with their brand and spend lots of money purchasing the testing strips that correspond to their particular monitors.

Third, they are quick. After sticking your finger, drawing a drop of blood, and applying it to the monitor, you typically have to wait only a total of five seconds to get the results. The only thing they have not yet achieved is absolute precision. They are not quite as accurate as we could wish they were. But they are getting better.

How Accurate Are Today's Blood Sugar Meters?

I did a test using four different blood sugar monitors to determine just how close they were to each other. For this experiment I used the Walgreens TRUE2go monitor, the FreeStyle Precision Neo, the FreeStyle Light, and the ReliOn Prime models. Testing myself in quick succession with the four monitors I came up with the following results.

FOUR GLUCOSE MONITOR MODELS USED IN RAPID SUCCESSION	
ReliOn Prime	118
FreeStyle Light	103
FreeStyle Precision Neo	96
Walgreens TRUE2go	88

Summary: Apparently not all glucose monitors are created equal. The short take to this little experiment: it's probably not a good idea to buy the cheapest model in the store!

I would have liked it so much more had all the monitors tested within about five points of each other. As it was, there was a 30-point difference between the highest number, 118, and the lowest, 88. That is a huge difference! The two cheapest monitors used were the ReliOn Prime (around $10) and the Walgreens TRUE2go (around $13). From what I know about my blood sugar levels as a result of a large numbers of tests, I felt these two monitors were the most inaccurate, with the Prime reading too high at 118 and the TRUE2go reading too low at 88. I would guess that my true blood was closer to the Neo or the FreeStyle Light readings of 96 or 103.

The takeaway from this simple experiment is this: The monitors you buy at your local discount store or drugstore are not perfect. You should have your doctor check your blood sugar shortly after you have taken your own blood sugar with your home monitor. If there is some disparity, and there almost surely will be, your doctor's number is the one you should accept. Second, you probably shouldn't buy the cheapest monitors in the store if you can help it. Go ahead and spend a few extra dollars and buy one that is a name brand and is slightly more expensive.

Testing Monitors Against Themselves

Later I decided I wanted to know how accurate blood sugar monitors would be when tested against themselves.

Testing Monitors Against Themselves

I took my two favorites, the FreeStyle Light and the FreeStyle Precision Neo, and tested myself once again in rapid succession. I was curious as to whether they could at least maintain consistency when compared with themselves a few seconds earlier or later.

FREESTYLE LIGHT SCORES IN RAPID SUCCESSION	
Test # 1	106
Test # 2	103
Test # 3	104
Test # 4	103

Summary: I was actually impressed with how close these scores were to each other. There was only a three-point difference between the highest number and the lowest. Pretty good!

FREESTYLE PRECISION NEO SCORES IN RAPID SUCCESSION	
Test # 1	111
Test # 2	108
Test # 3	109
Test # 4	107
Summary: Like its more expensive brother, the Precision Neo did well in measuring itself against itself. It only had a four-point difference from the highest to the lowest score.	

Basics of Testing

The first question we will consider concerning blood-glucose testing is the why. Until the why question is settled, the how and the when don't really mean much. We human beings are naturally partly selfish and partly pragmatic in the choices we make. We tend to do the things we consider either pleasurable or valuable to us. And there is nothing particularly pleasurable about sticking your fingers over and over again with a sharp little needle (at least not for normal people). So the pleasure angle is definitely out.

The other motivating factor has to do with value. Is blood sugar testing of any real value to the diabetic or the prediabetic? The answer to this question is an emphatic, definite, positive, absolute "Yes!" Testing your blood sugar is incredibly valuable. To illustrate this, let us consider the game of golf.

I have always loved golf, although I've never been very good at it. But whatever skills I have, I owe to my trips to the driving range, where golfers hit ball after ball in search of the perfect swing. It is not enough just to hit one or two good shots over the course of nine or eighteen holes. The goal is to swing well consistently, which is about the most difficult challenge found in any sport for most of us hackers.

Feedback!

Still, even hackers can improve their swing and their game as a result of hours spent at the driving range. The reason this tends to help is due to feedback. The idea is this: Let's say as you practice hitting golf balls, you hit a terrible golf shot that starts out way right and ends up farther right and out of bounds. As you watch the little golf ball sizzling its way to nowhere, you say to yourself, "This is not the way I want my golf shots to go! My swing was off. I am going to have to do something different." You make changes. You change your tempo or your grip or your stance or whatever changes you feel need to be made and try again. When you find yourself hitting a solid shot that goes fairly straight, and then find you can follow up that shot with another good one, and then another, you know you are on the right track. You are doing something right, or in the case of golf, you are likely doing several things right.

Your eyes play a large role in this. When you see the ball going where you do not want it to go, you know that changes are called for. But when you see the ball flying 250 yards down the center, you figure this is a swing worth attempting to repeat. This is why when a golfer hits a shot, he does not continue to look down at the ground. He doesn't turn around and talk to his buddy. As soon as the swing is complete, he looks carefully to see where the ball went. Good shot: Don't mess with anything. Bad shot: Don't do that again!

Feedback is all important. If you went to a driving range and hit balls blindfolded, you would be defeating the purpose. You wouldn't know whether your shots were good, bad, or mediocre. You couldn't make the necessary adjustments, and your game would never improve.

What does this have to do with diabetes? Everything! Just like the golfer needs feedback to see whether he did well or poorly, and make adjustments to his swing, so the diabetic and the prediabetic require feedback to gain an understanding of how well they are doing with the foods they regularly eat.

And that is where your friendly little blood sugar monitor is invaluable. It gives you instant feedback. If you don't use a monitor, you are like the golfer who is at the driving range hitting golf balls with a blindfold over his eyes. You will have no clue whether you are eating well or poorly, whether you are driving your blood sugar levels off the charts or keeping them under control. Nor will you ever be motivated to make any real, significant changes in your diet that could save your health and your life. You will be in the dark, and you will stay in the dark.

It is not difficult. If you eat a meal, and one hour later your monitor reads 95, you know you have just hit a beautiful drive 250 yards down the center of the fairway. If it reads 180, you have clearly mis-hit the ball and pushed it into the trees. And if it jumps up over 200, you have dumped your ball into the lake.

To sum up, your blood sugar monitor is your friend. You had better learn to love it, use it, and if you don't have one, run to the drugstore or discount store and buy one without delay. It will give you the feedback you need to know how you are doing and how the meals you are eating are affecting your body.

Common Tests

I have been primarily talking about testing with a glucose monitor that you can purchase nearly everywhere, but you should be aware that this is not the only type of test that relates to diabetes. Four of the most common blood sugar tests are:

1. The A1C Test

2. The Glucose Tolerance Test

3. The Fasting Blood Sugar Test

4. The Post-Meal Test

The A1C test is a very good test, and it determines your average blood sugar level over the course of the previous two or three months. More and more doctors are leaning on this test to diagnose diabetes. It won't give you numbers like your glucose monitor does, such as 95, 130, 180, and so forth. It will give you numbers like 5.5 or 6.4 or 7.6, or higher. There are charts that can translate these A1C numbers into an average blood sugar level number such as you would see on your home monitor. But doctors break down A1C numbers like this:

- 5.6 or Lower: Normal
- 5.7–6.4: Prediabetic
- 6.5 or Higher: Diabetic

For most prediabetics, keeping our A1C somewhere in the 5 range is desirable. The low 6s are problematic; the high 6s are diabetic. And if your A1C is 7 or higher, you have real problems. It is a great test and is a surer "report card" than the fasting blood sugar score you get with a common glucose monitor. It used to be that you could only get this kind of a test from a doctor, but these days A1C tests are often available in many stores, although ideally you should have it done at a doctor's office. The physycian can help you interpret the score and establish a plan of action to improve your next test. The one weakness of this test is that it doesn't give you any information at all about particular foods and meals you may be eating. If you are eating vegetable salads every other night for dinner, and spaghetti with French bread and with apple pie and ice cream on the alternating nights, you never would know by this test which of the meals were helpful and which were harmful to blood sugar. If your score is too high, the most you could learn would be that you definitely have blood sugar issues. But what to do, what to change, what to eliminate…you would have no clue.

Personal A1C Test

I purchased a ReliOn A1C test from Walmart and gave it a try. Sometime before, a doctor had given me an A1C test, and it had revealed a score of 5.8. Amazingly, when I did the ReliOn test at home, it read 5.9. You could hardly ask for more accuracy than that! The 5.8–5.9 range is good, but it is not great. It is not a diabetic number, but it does indicate prediabetes, which is where I have been testing for years. Would I prefer it in the low 5s? Sure I would, but the fact that I have been able to keep full-scale diabetes at bay for the last 17 years, by the grace of God, is no small thing to me, and I am very, very grateful.

The glucose tolerance test, ideally administered by a diabetes specialist, determines quite precisely whether you have insulin resistance. After an eight-hour period without food, a sugary sweet drink is administered. Blood sugar is tested at various intervals, with a priority given to the test conducted at the two-hour mark. By this time a person without diabetes should have their blood sugar below 140 mg/dl. And at no time should a nondiabetic have their blood sugar rise above 200. If you have both of these symptoms, a blood sugar rise above 200 and your blood sugar still over 140 two hours later, you are considered likely to have diabetes. This test was once the gold standard for determining diabetes, but these days two consecutive A1C scores of 6.5 or higher are considered a more certain indicator of diabetes.

The glucose tolerance test is a good test for determining whether you have blood sugar problems, no doubt about it. But like the A1C test, it does nothing to indicate which foods or meals may be giving you problems. It gives you no hint about what changes you ought to make. In the past many doctors simply tested you, determined if you were diabetic, and then on that basis either prescribed or didn't prescribe an oral agent or insulin. If your score was too high, you got medication or insulin; if it was acceptable, you didn't. They might tell you to "take it easy on the sweets," but that was the extent of the counsel from most doctors in those days. Not exactly a proactive approach to conquering diabetes!

The fasting blood sugar test can also indicate diabetes, although few doctors rely on this alone. It simply involves testing your blood sugar in the morning after going through the night without eating or drinking anything but water. It is a fairly decent report card on how you have been doing. Someone with insulin resistance who is paying no attention to what he eats and is loading himself with carbs will nearly always have a higher than normal fasting blood sugar level. The current line of demarcation between diabetic and nondiabetic is 126. If you can go all night without eating and then wake up in the morning, test yourself, and see a score of 130, 140, or above, you can be pretty sure you are diabetic. You should not depend on one test alone, however. You would need to see a consistent pattern of high numbers.

By now you can probably guess what I am about to say. Like the other tests, this also does not give you any indication about which dietary rules you may be breaking—what got you in this place in the first place. In some ways this is like going to a doctor, who examines you and then says, "You're in terrible shape!" When you grill him about what got you that way or what you can do to improve your health, he gives you no answer. He simply keeps shaking his head and muttering, "You're a mess. You're really a mess." Perhaps the best response to such a doctor would be to get up in his face and shout, "Okay, I got it. I'm a mess! But why am I a mess? How did I get to be such a mess? And what can I do to stop being a mess?"

I guess you could say that the doctor has done you a favor, but not much of one. It's not enough to know we have problems. Those of us with insulin resistance and diabetic glucose levels desperately need to know how we got that way and what practical steps we can take to lead us out of the mess. And that brings us to the fourth test.

The post-meal glucose test is the one test that not only indicates blood sugar problems but gives us powerful insight about what we can do to remedy the situation. It is not a general test that merely measures our level of impairment; it is a very specific test. It reveals the tendency of specific foods to raise our blood sugar. It reveals which foods and meals are gentle with our blood sugar levels and which ones are dangerous and potentially lethal (over time). The great news is that this is a test we can do on ourselves at any time, in almost any place, in a matter of under a minute. When we go to Walmart or Walgreens or our local grocery store and spend our $15 on a glucose monitor and another $20 on a package of 50 test strips, we now have in our hands the means by which we can start making powerful changes that can totally turn things around for us, day by day and meal by meal. If we will listen to our little blood sugar monitor and embrace his wisdom, we will see all those numbers on the other tests start to come down. Our fasting blood sugar will slowly and surely decrease, as will our A1C scores. Out of the darkness and into the light!

As we have indicated, this test involves eating a specific food or meal, noting carefully what you have eaten (and drunk), waiting a period of time, and then testing ourselves when our blood sugar levels are typically peaking. Blood sugar peaks can differ from one individual to the next, so there is really no set time that fits everyone. Typically, the worse your insulin resistance and the weaker your pancreas, the longer it will take your blood sugar to peak and then come down. Because I was able to make changes before I blew out my pancreas, it still works pretty well despite my insulin resistance, and I find I normally peak around one hour after I finish eating. Beans and pasta tend to create more of a delay, so with them I sometimes wait an hour and 15 minutes or an hour and a half. By testing yourself in 15-minute intervals between an hour and two hours after several meals, you should be able to determine the proper interval of time you should allow to elapse between finishing your meal and testing yourself.

How to Test Yourself

Blood sugar monitoring kits normally consist of three main parts: the monitor itself, a lancing device for piercing your finger in order to obtain a drop of blood, and testing strips. These kits will usually include several "lancets," which are tiny little needles housed in plastic bodies and used inside the lancing device. When you first try out your lancing device, you might find that it doesn't sting and creates no blood drop. This is because these devices do not come with a needle inside. You will have to insert one of the lancets into the device for it to work. Remove the top from your lancing device and place one of the lancets in the open cavity, lining up the ridges in the lancets with the grooves in the lancing device. Twist off the round "head" exposing the needle. Replace the top of the lancing device and you are ready to go.

Take a testing strip and place it in the monitor. The strips have metal contacts that must be inserted "head-first" into the monitor. It does matter which side goes up. If you have inserted the strip correctly, you will see an image of a blood drop appear in a few seconds, telling you that the monitor has been activated and the testing strip is ready to receive a drop of blood.

Set the monitor down and pick up your lancing device. This device will have an adjustment wheel that will show several different numbers. By adjusting the numbers, you are determining how deeply the needle will pierce your fingers. Set the number low at first. No use piercing yourself any deeper than necessary. If that number doesn't provide a nice drop of blood, you may have to set the number higher. For most people 2 or 3 will be satisfactory.

The typical lancing device must be cocked, sort of like a gun. You do this by holding the base of the device with one hand and pulling back on the rear with the other. With the device cocked and set to the proper level, place it up on the edge of one of your fingers or your thumb. Either hand will work. Normally I don't use my little finger as it has the least blood in it. Make sure the lancing device is squarely up against your finger. Press the little button to release the needle to do its job and pierce your finger. Once you've done this, set your lancing device down and give your finger a squeeze to force a drop of blood to appear on the skin. With your other hand, pick up your monitor and place the testing strip against the drop of blood. Your monitor will either give you a beep or some visual signal on its face to let you know that it has received enough blood. Immediately take the strip away from your finger. With most monitors, all you have to do is wait for five seconds to get your results. And that's all there is to it. It's quick, easy, highly informative, and relatively painless.

Problems with Testing

Once you've been doing this often, this will be no problem at all, but in the early days you may have some trouble. In my experience there are two reasons why novices have so much trouble getting their monitors to work for them: 1) They are nervous about sticking themselves and do not press the lancing device firmly against their fingers. Thinking they are saving themselves a little pain, they are simply short-circuiting the process and will have to do it again and again, and 2) they have not yet figured out the proper squeezing procedure. Usually that blood drop will not appear until you give your finger a squeeze. I do this by using a thumb-thumb-forefinger-surround method. Using the thumb of the hand on which the finger has been pierced, plus my other thumb and forefinger, I surround the area pierced and squeeze from three sides. A decent-sized blood drop nearly always appears.

No soldier would go out to a battle without a rifle in his hand. No baseball player would walk up to the plate without a bat. No golfer would go out to the golf course without any golf clubs. And no sensible diabetic or prediabetic would attempt to fight the terrible foe of diabetes without making frequent use of their blood sugar monitor.

Testing my blood sugar has long been a normal part of my life. I don't always do it every day, mainly because I have tested myself so often and for so long that I have a pretty good idea what most foods and meals will do to my blood sugar levels. But when I try out new foods or new combinations of foods, I will bring out my old friend and put him to good use. And sometimes I will test myself on a food or a meal that I have already tested in the past, just to see if anything has changed.

A Day in My Life

To demonstrate the value of testing, I decided to administer post-meal blood sugar tests after each of my meals for a single day. On this particular Thursday I recorded my blood sugar before each meal and one hour after each meal. The meals were ones that were fairly common to me: eggs and bacon, with toast (made from the lowest-carb bread in the local stores—7 net grams of carbs) and low-carb jelly. For some vitamin C, I added a mandarin (like a tiny orange—about 8 grams of carbs). For lunch I had a tuna sandwich with two slices of the same 7-net-carb-grams-per-slice bread and added a small sugar-free yogurt.

For dinner I really treated myself. I had a pizza and chocolate cake! Now, before you become shocked, let me explain. The pizza was made with two low-carb tortilla shells (5 net grams of carbs each). The topping ingredients were all fairly low-carb, so the pizza was not likely to do serious damage to my blood sugar. But what about the chocolate cake? The cake was a homemade concoction (approximately 6 net grams carbs).

Ingredients: 1 egg, 1 T. of Carbquik (an extremely low-carb baking mix), 1 T. of almond flour (also very low-carb), 1 tsp. of unsweetened cocoa, 2 T. of Stevia, a couple of shakes of salt, 1 ½ tsp. of baking powder, 1 tsp. of sour cream, 1 small sugar-free chocolate bar cut into tiny bits, and a handful of almond slices.

Directions: Spray a large mug with cooking spray. Place all the ingredients in the mug and stir vigorously until all is well-blended. Place in microwave for about 95 seconds.

I get a kick out of eating foods and meals that would make people who know what I advocate think I was the biggest hypocrite in the world if they saw me eating them. But in truth I was staying low-carb while eating wonderful foods that tasted great. I was pretty sure that the combination of pizza and chocolate cake would not be much of a problem, but still there are always some surprises.

My breakfast of eggs, bacon, and relatively low-carb toast proved the least trouble to my pancreas. My pre-test revealed a 105, and my peak, if you want to call it that, was 104. So an hour after breakfast, my blood sugar was essentially the same as before. I have no problem with that!

After my lunch of a tuna sandwich and sugar-free yogurt, my blood sugar jumped from 108 to 126. This was a bit higher than I expected, but still, when you peak in the 120s, you are doing pretty well.

By suppertime my blood sugar had dropped to 99. I really enjoyed the pizza and chocolate cake. I put some whipped cream on top of the cake because whipped cream is surprisingly low in sugar. This was the meal I was most curious about. I had never tested this combination before. An hour after eating, my blood sugar peak was 117, an 18-point rise.

I was one happy guy. I had gone an entire day with relatively normal blood sugar. Here was a day I was not harming my body with excessively high blood sugar. If I do the same the next day, and the next, week after week, month after month, and year after year, I can work my way through life unlikely to experience the terrible complications of diabetes and runaway blood sugar.

A DAY IN MY LIFE			
	BREAKFAST Eggs, Bacon, Low-Carb Toast, Mandarin	LUNCH Tuna Sandwich, Sugar-Free Yogurt	DINNER Low-Carb Pizza, Low-Carb Cake
Before Eating	105	108	99
After 1 Hour	104	126	117
Total Blood sugar Rise	-1 mg/dl	18 mg/dl	18 mg/dl

Summary: My pre-test numbers were not great. Normal people will usually test in the 80s or at most the low 90s when they haven't eaten for several hours. My fasting blood sugar of 105 in the morning was surely an indication that I have some blood sugar issues. Still, I was able to keep my blood sugar levels "inbounds" throughout the day by making wise food choices, even without taking any oral medications or insulin. I was especially delighted to be able to eat homemade pizza and chocolate cake and find that my blood sugar never even reached 120!

Pizza Tests

While most of the tests in this book are tests I have done on myself, I have endeavored to enlist a few "guinea pigs" to be test subjects here and there. One of these is my old friend David Dryden. Dave and I served together as elders in a church in north Texas years ago, and he has been on my board since I founded Spirit of Grace Ministries. When Dave's doctor first told him he was a type 2 diabetic, it was a great shock to him. He had never imagined he would ever be diabetic. He wasn't overweight and was conscientious about his health. At the time of his diagnosis, his A1C score was running at 6.8. These days it has worsened a bit and is normally around 7.2. Dave is no predia-betic; he is a genuine, full-fledged type 2 diabetic. At first, he tried to control his diabetes with diet and exercise alone, but now he takes oral medication.

Blood Sugar Testing with an Old Friend

Dave agreed to test himself with pizza. First, we went to a local pizza restaurant and enjoyed pizza the way most people do. We ate five slices of medium-crust pizza along with a small token salad and drank regular soda to wash it down. The meal certainly tasted great, and afterward we went back to Dave's house to wait for one hour to elapse and then checked his blood sugar.

His pre-test blood sugar was remarkably low. It has been at 76 mg/dl. The medication he was taking was definitely helping out. After one hour his blood sugar has risen dramatically—all the way to 281, over a 200-point rise! I also tested myself before and one hour after and had eaten the exact same meal. In my case, my blood sugar jumped from 99 to 172, a 73-point rise.

About a week later Dave and I went back to the same restaurant. This time we modified our meal to make it significantly lower in carbs. It was by no means a low-carb meal, but it was definitely a lower-carb meal than previously. This time we ate four pieces of thin-crust pizza. We ate a larger salad, and we drank diet sodas rather than regular. Again, we went back to his house, waited until an hour had elapsed since we finished the meal, and tested ourselves.

Dave's pre-meal test revealed a 93, again a very good number, espe-cially for a diabetic. After the thin-crust pizza, the larger salad, and the diet drink, his one-hour post-meal test showed him at 178—an 85-point rise. It was not as low as I had hoped it would be, but still, he had shaved off a lot of points. An 85-point rise beats a 200-point rise! When I asked Dave what he thought he might do to get those numbers even lower, he hit the nail right on the proverbial head: "Less pizza and more salad." In my case, the post-meal test was wonderful. After a pre-meal test of 100, my blood sugar peaked at 113, a little 13-point rise. Clearly, as a prediabetic I could get away with more than Dave could.

MEDIUM-CRUST PIZZA WITH REGULAR SODA TEST		
	David	Dennis
Before Eating	76	99
After 1 Hour	281	172
Total Blood sugar Rise	205 mg/dl	73 mg/dl

Summary: I knew our blood sugar levels would rise significantly, and they surely did. However, I didn't expect that Dave's would rise as high as it did. He and I were both surprised. This is not a meal he should be eating ever again!

THIN-CRUST PIZZA WITH DIET SODA TEST		
	David	Dennis
Before Eating	93	100
After 1 Hour	178	113
Total Blood Sugar Rise	85 mg/dl	13 mg/dl

Summary: I thought Dave would do better than he did on this one. Peaking at 178, he was still in an unhealthy place, blood sugar–wise. My peak of 113 was surprisingly good, considering I had just eaten four pieces of pizza. The thin crust made the difference. These two tests reveal three simple but important insights: 1) Some people can tolerate more carbs than others, 2) the amount of bread you put in your mouth makes an enormous difference, and 3) whatever you may say about artificially sweetened diet sodas, they clearly do not affect blood sugar the way sugar-laden sodas do.

Tests like these are so very important. I could have "preached" to Dave about the importance of avoiding a lot of bread and laying off regular sodas. But preaching is just so… preachy. It often stirs up the rebel in us and moves us to do the very opposite of the message preached. But in this case, I didn't have to do much preaching. Dave's own blood sugar monitor did all the preaching, just as my blood sugar monitors have been gently but firmly preaching to me for years. And somehow I can tolerate preaching from my monitor, which is not biased and speaks rather quietly. I find it much easier to accept than the "preaching" I get from living people, even the so-called experts (who often oppose each other). My $20 monitor is a nice, honest, nonthreatening little fella, and I have kept diabetes at bay for a good long while by listening to him.

Who's the Boss?

Do you remember when you were a kid, and your older brother or sister would try to boss you around. You probably said something like, "You're not the boss of me!" You might put up with your momma telling you what to do, but you weren't about to allow your sibling to act like Momma. But when it comes to eating for the diabetic or the prediabetic, your blood sugar monitor really ought to be the "boss of you." You need to allow it to tell you what you can eat and what you cannot eat; what is acceptable and what is strictly off-limits. And any food or combination of foods that sends your blood sugar soaring to 180, 200, 230, and beyond will have to be either eliminated from your diet or modified or reduced to much smaller portions until your blood sugar stays at a reasonable level. Author and diabetes expert Jenny Ruhl calls this "eating to the meter."[2] She writes, "What you're doing when you 'eat to your meter' is creating a low-spike diet rather than a low-carbohydrate diet."[3]

The way I interpret this is that it means we are not necessarily overly concerned with how many carbs we are eating at any one meal. The answer will be different from one individual to the next and from one meal to the next. But if, by the meals and foods we choose, we can keep our blood sugar from peaking any higher than our target limit (and for me that limit is 140 mg/dl), and we do this meal after meal and day after day, it is extremely likely that our fasting blood sugar will go down, our A1C number will go down, and we'll be on our way to a lifetime of good health and normal blood sugar.

3

Check Those Labels!

Nutritional labels have been around for a long time, and most people today cannot remember a time when packaged foods on the grocery store shelves didn't have some kind of nutritional label on them. However, standardized and easy-to-read labels made their debut in the early 1990s. They have been evolving since then. Before the reformation and standardization of labels in the '90s, the labels varied greatly and could be extremely confusing. Dr. Louis Sullivan, who played a major role in making nutritional labels what they are today, said at that time, "The grocery store has become a *Tower of Babel* and consumers need to be linguists, scientists and mind readers to understand the many labels they see."[1]

Things have changed since then, and nutritional labels today are simple and to the point. You can see at a glance the calories, carbs, and protein amounts in the food, along with the major vitamins. One area of confusion that remains has to do with serving size, but we'll get to that.

In my early days as a prediabetic I didn't concern myself with labels too much. Once I understood that my high blood sugar levels were largely a product of eating high-carb foods, I made a reasonable decision: I quit eating high-carb foods, and in those cases where I felt socially compelled to eat them, I ate them in small quantities. But for the most part I paid a lot more attention to the numbers on my blood sugar monitor than the numbers on nutritional labels. In time, however, I had a revelation: the amount of carbs on the nutritional labels of foods could be used to predict my blood sugar levels. Once I realized that, I began looking more closely and more often at the nutritional labels of foods on the grocery shelves.

Inspect Those Labels!

As you look at a nutritional label, there are four important listings to which diabetics need to give special attention. First, obviously, check out the total carbs. For diabetics, carbohydrates are about a zillion times more important than calories. People who reduce their carbohydrates significantly typically don't struggle too much with weight anyway, but our great focus must always be on blood sugar, and blood sugar is inevitably and irreversibly linked to the carbs we ingest. Before granting a food permission to take its place on our plate, we want to know not how pretty it is, not how much vitamin C it contains, not how many or how few calories it contains, not whether it is higher in protein or fat, but "how many carbs is this food going to cost me?" We must be cheapies when it comes to carbs. We must not be willing to overspend on carbs, just for the privilege of indulging in a baked potato or a slice of apple pie a la mode. We truly cannot afford it!

But there is another listing on the nutritional label that is almost as important as the total amount of carbs, and that is the serving size. If you do not check out the serving size, you can easily be deceived. For example, one can of soup declares it has 22 grams of carbohydrate. That doesn't sound too bad. But when you check out the serving size, you find that all the numbers listed pertain to half the can. And since nearly everybody would eat the entire can of soup, you will have to double the carbohydrates to get an accurate reflection of how many carbs this soup will cost you. While 22 grams of soup isn't so bad, 44 grams is a lot. Regular candy bars contain around 33 grams of carbs, and sodas contain about 40. So when you eat this can of soup, you are getting more carbs (which will rapidly convert to sugar) than you would if you ate a candy bar or drank a soda. Granted, they may not spike your blood sugar quite as fast, but do not suppose that those 44 grams of soup carbs are inconsequential to your blood sugar.

A small bottle of Nesquik chocolate milk lists 24 grams of carbs, again not such a scary number. But let your eyes go up the label a bit and you find that this only represents half the bottle, so in reality when you drink that small bottle of chocolate milk, you'll be ingesting a whopping 48 grams of carbs—more than a regular-sized candy bar and more than most 12-ounce sodas.

Fiber Is Your Friend

The next listing that is vital for diabetics to consider is the dietary fiber. Fiber is a carb, but it is the one carb that typically does not increase blood sugar. Your body gives it a free pass and makes no attempt to convert this type of carb into sugar. The fiber simply passes through your body without doing any harm. In fact, it does good, as it helps keep your colon flushed out and cleaned up (at least as clean as a colon can be!).

What this means is that when you see foods that have fiber listed as a subset of their carbs, you can deduct the fiber from the total carbs to see what this food will truly do to raise your blood sugar. A good example of this is the avocado. An avocado is not really a low-carb food. One cup of sliced avocado has 12 grams of carbs. That's not too high, but it's not low either. However, out of those 12 carb grams, 10 of them come from fiber and will have no effect on your blood sugar. So an avocado is not at all likely to significantly raise your blood sugar.

Flaxseed meal is a food that is almost all fiber. Two cups of flaxseed contain 97 grams of carbs. But all but five of those carbs are fiber carbs, so you could put 2 cups of flaxseed meal into something you cook, and you would have almost no net carbs to deal with from the flaxseed. The essential formula for determining carbs is this:

Total Carbohydrate
- Dietary Fiber
_____

Net Carbs (the carbs that raise blood sugar)

Don't Be Impressed!

As you look at the packaging of foods, by all means be impressed when you see a low-carbohydrate number on the label or when you discover that the majority of the carbs in a food are fiber carbs. But there are some boasts that you should not be duped by when you see them proudly displayed on the packaging. First, you should not be impressed by the term *gluten-free*. That simply means that the food contains no wheat, barley, or rye. This is really inconsequential to the diabetic or prediabetic. A huge bowl of rice, for example, is gluten-free, but it spells disaster for your blood sugar. Corn Flakes are gluten-free, but if you think your body is going to be impressed and your blood sugar will behave itself, think again. The idea of going gluten-free has become fashionable these days, but it means little unless you happen to be allergic to wheat. But if that's not your case, don't go looking for gluten-free foods and suppose you are solving your blood sugar problems.

Other terms that should not impress you are *fat-free* and *low fat*. In fact, not only should you not be impressed, you really ought to be scared when you see these words proudly displayed on food packaging. Because in nearly every case, when food companies make a food product fat-free or low fat, they make up for the lack of taste with added sugar. Nearly every time you compare a fat-free or low-fat food to the original food, the reduced-fat food is higher in sugar and will create far more trouble for your blood sugar levels. For people who struggle with runaway blood sugar, their problem is not fat; it's carbohydrates. Fat doesn't even budge your blood sugar upward the least bit, but carbs, especially refined and processed carbs, will send it soaring!

When Free Is Not So Free

A great example of fat-free versus regular may be found in the Kraft Ranch salad dressing. The classic version of Kraft Ranch dressing has 2 grams of carbs per 2 tablespoons—about as low as you're going to find in salad dressings. But when you check out the fat-free version, you find that the carbs have been bumped up from 2 to 11 grams. Because most people are going to use a lot more than 2 tablespoons of dressing on a larger salad, they will be getting 22 or perhaps 33 grams of carbs from their fat-free dressing alone! The Kraft folks added sugar and who knows what else to their fat-free dressing to make up for the tasteless-ness that always occurs when you remove the fat. Unsuspecting, naive people, seeing the fat-free label, will choose this version, thinking they are doing themselves a favor. They are not.

Another deceptive term is *cholesterol-free*. So what if a food is cho-lesterol-free? Every non-animal-based food is cholesterol-free. Dough-nuts, depending on how they're fried, can be cholesterol-free. Many sugary cereals are cholesterol-free. Potato chips are cholesterol-free, but this by no means makes them good for you. You are far better off eat-ing some grilled chicken or a couple of eggs than gorging on a bag of cholesterol-free potato chips.

The next terms I want to mention are going to shock you, but I have to say it: Don't be overly impressed with *whole wheat* or *whole grain*. Now, I know some of you are already shouting, "Blasphemy!" and call-ing me a food heretic. But please hear me out before tossing this book in the trash. Here's what I mean. Whole grain foods are indeed pref-erable to their white cousins. So if you are determined to eat a piece of bread, by all means choose whole grain bread over white. If you must eat rice, go for brown over white. The extra fiber and extra nutrition will help…somewhat.

But do not suppose that just because a food is whole grain it gets a free pass when it comes to its effect upon your blood sugar. Brown rice and white rice are nearly identical in total carbs. The extra fiber will probably slow down your blood sugar spike a bit, but you will get a spike nonetheless. Don't become so excited about the term *whole grain* that you assume you can eat as much whole grain bread, whole grain cereal, and whole grain rice as your heart desires. You definitely cannot if you have insulin resistance and really want to achieve nor-mal blood sugar levels. (We'll look at this a little more closely later in the book.)

Be a Carb-Saver

When checking out nutritional labels, one rule of thumb that I use is what I call the Snickers bar comparison. One regular Snickers candy bar contains around 33 grams of carbs. So when I'm looking at a nutritional label and see that this food has between 30 to 35 grams of carbs, I say to myself, *That's about like eating a Snickers bar!* If I see a food that has between 60 to 70 grams of carbs, I say, *That's like eating two Snickers bars!* Now, eating an entire dinner that includes quite a bit of fiber and has around 30 grams of carbs total would probably work for me, but eating one small food item that rapidly pours 30 grams of carbs into my bloodstream most definitely doesn't.

Let's consider the difference between generic versus standard versions of various items you can purchase in your discount store. A while back I took a look at two antacids that both contained the exact amount of the same active ingredient, 750 milligrams of calcium carbonate. The Tums version cost more than $4, whereas the generic version, which was identical in what it could do for you, cost less than $2. So why would anybody spend more than $4 for something when you could get the precise equivalent for less than $2?

The point I'm making is that, unless you are independently wealthy, it would be better for most of us to go with the cheaper version. And when it comes to carbohydrates and food, I have to have that same attitude. Why would I want to eat something high carb when I could get something similar that is low carb? Why eat tacos with a 25-carb-gram shell when I could easily purchase low-carb shells that contain only 5 net grams of carbs? Why eat a huge stack of pancakes smothered with sugar-laden syrup, which will absolutely overwhelm my body's blood sugar processing system, when I could eat a stack of low-carb, almond flour pancakes with a few strawberries on top? Or have eggs, bacon, and a low-carb muffin, which will hardly budge my blood sugar?

I know people must think I am weird (and they're probably not too far off), but I will sometimes linger at a particular area of the store, checking out the carbs and fiber for every brand of a particular food product for carbs and fiber. This helps me make wise choices. I do not make my purchase based on price or any particular brand name. I don't care a thing about calories. I am looking exclusively for the lowest number I can find when I deduct fiber from total carbs for a realistic serving size of that particular food. When I find one brand of food with a significantly lower net-carb gram number than all the others, I feel as if I have hit the jackpot.

The Produce Section

Food found in your produce section will not contain nutrition information. God didn't see fit to put nutrition facts on oranges, carrots, and spinach leaves, and neither have the grocers, although if the produce is prepackaged, it will probably have that information on the bag. Of course, you can look up the carbs and fiber in virtually every fruit or vegetable on the internet, and I have often done this. But one general rule is simply this: Most vegetables are safe, and most fruits are not so safe. Once again, I face stoning from the naturalists who feel that anything that grows out of the ground is wonderful and anything that comes from a dead animal is horrible, horrible, horrible. Thus, in their minds, to dare to suggest that fruit may be even the slightest bit problematic is dietary folly of the worst kind.

But there is one thing you have to remember: My firm convictions about safe and not-so-safe foods come directly from one fundamental source: my blood sugar monitor. No matter how natural, no matter how colorful, no matter how organic, no matter how many nutritionists go on and on about the vitamins a food may contain, if my blood sugar monitor tells me it's a problem for me, then it's a problem for me. And in case you say, "Well, you're not a doctor or a nutritionist. You're just a simpleton," I must remind you that Dr. Richard Bernstein, perhaps the premiere diabetic doctor in the United States, who is himself a type 1 diabetic, has come to the exact same conclusion. I saw him in a video mentioning that he has not eaten fruit for some 20 years.[2] Apparently his blood sugar monitor and my blood sugar monitor are saying the same exact thing: The natural sugar in fruit can spell big troubles for diabetics.

Here's something to ponder: fruits taste sweet and most vegetables do not (carrots and sugar snap peas are some exceptions). Why do you suppose this is? It is because fruits have far more sugar than vegetables. Somehow the majority of Americans have fallen for the myth that states that natural sugar is entirely harmless and has no effect on glucose levels. Wrong! The sugar in fruit may spike less than the sugar in a candy bar, but it will still raise your blood sugar. A nondiabetic may very well be able to eat several fruits and still have great blood sugar levels, but that proves exactly nothing. In this book I am not talking about nondiabetics; I am talking about people whose blood sugar mechanisms have been severely impaired. And a key aspect of that impairment is the inability to process sugar, period—whether it comes from chocolate cake or apple pie, or oranges, pineapples, or bananas. If someone put a gun to my head and said I must eat either a big piece of chocolate cake or a large apple and a banana, I would choose the fruit over the cake, for sure. But in all my years, no one has ever forced me at the point of a gun to eat either of those, and I have a strong suspicion I will likely finish my years on this earth without that ever happening to me!

This being said, my diet is not entirely fruit-free. I do eat berries, which are a kinder, gentler version of fruit than most of the others. And sometimes I will have half an apple at a meal that is otherwise very low in carbs. I am not on a crusade to get all people everywhere to forsake fruit. But I am saying, "Be a bit careful!"

Taco Delight

To demonstrate the value of checking the carbs, I set up a blood sugar taco test for myself. To make sure I got the best bang for my buck, I went to the store and checked out every hard taco shell brand they sold. I discovered that the La Tierra taco shells had a mere 4 grams of carbs per shell. This meant, if my math skills haven't failed me, that I would only be getting 12 grams of carbs from three taco shells. Of course, I would be filling the shells with hamburger meat, lettuce, shredded cheese, and tomatoes, and then I'd put some picante sauce on top of each taco. So all these ingredients would add to the carb count, but none of them would be very high in carbs.

Three Tacos Plus Avocado Test

I estimated that three tacos might cost me a little over 20 grams of carbs. From previous tests I know that normally I can tolerate meals that have up to 30 grams of carbs. So unless some strange phenomenon occurred, my blood sugar monitor should yield a friendly number on my post-meal test. I did drink a diet soda with the tacos because taco meals somehow seem incomplete without soda. I know by experience that diet sodas tend to make my blood sugar go down rather than up, so I wasn't worried about that.

There was one problem with this meal. Three of these small tacos probably would not fill me up. I would need another food. One of the standard add-ons to Mexican foods is chips, but that was out. Instead, I added a small avocado. Avocados are one of God's gifts to diabetics. Here was a filler food that was not going to break the bank (the blood sugar bank, that is).

My pre-meal test was at 91, which was a good number for me. One hour after finishing the three tacos and avocado, my blood sugar had risen to a scrawny little 104. This represented a 13-point rise, which made me exceedingly happy. You may ask, "If I eat the same meal, will I get similar results?" No, I can't promise that, but I can tell you that you will definitely see lower numbers with these tacos than you would with three 25-carb-grams tacos. Try this yourself. Eat the identical meal, test yourself before and one hour after eating, and see how your body responds.

TACO TEST	
	Three 4-Grams-Carbs Taco Shells Plus Avocado
Before Eating	91
After 1 Hour	104
Total Blood sugar Rise	13 mg/dl

Summary: I get a strange delight in eating meals that most people suppose should be off-limits for diabetics while knowing that they are in truth low carb and will barely raise my blood sugar. Here is yet another food that many might suppose would be off the menu for me, and yet with the right brand of taco shells, I can have it! As for the high-carb taco shells, thanks, but no thanks.

Eric Cooper

I get many, many emails from people who have read my books on blood sugar and are seeing wonderful results. One of the most powerful of these emails was from a man named Eric Cooper. His reports on his blood sugar levels were so glowing and he had such enthusiasm that I asked him if I could come to his house (he is a fellow Texan) and interview him about his experience with conquering runaway blood sugar. He graciously agreed, and so on a rainy morning my wife, Benedicta, and I made the drive to Eric's house. When we arrived, we found Eric and his wife, Deborah, to be a delightful couple, and boy, did Eric ever have a story to tell!

Before we got around to the interview, they served us a wonderful low-carb lunch consisting of a salad and chicken soup, which had many vegetables but zero rice, noodles, or corn starch. It was a delicious meal, and we tested our blood sugar levels before we ate and then after we finished the interview, about an hour later. Both of us had good numbers, and Eric's blood sugar peaked at the one-hour mark at 125—which was lower than his typical fasting blood sugar had been six months ago! Clearly, he had made a lot of progress in a short time.

After the meal we sat down in a couple of comfortable chairs and talked. Eric told me that he had been retired for five years at that point and that his blood sugar problems seemed to develop after retirement, perhaps as a result of a less active lifestyle and gaining some weight. Eric had been conscientious to get check-ups with his doctor, and prior to retirement his blood sugar numbers were decent. Over several years of retirement living, his fasting blood sugar levels and his A1C scores crept steadily higher.

Finally, his doctor told him that if his A1C gained one more tenth of a point she would have to put him on insulin, a thought that scared Eric to death. Suddenly he gained tremendous motivation to do something about his blood sugar situation, but at the beginning he said he did "all the wrong things." He bought diabetic cookbooks and read various articles, but he stated, "Everything we read sent us in the wrong direction, because there was little to no improvement. The drop in my A1C was minimal."

Some diabetic writings pushed the value of whole wheat bread, so Eric was having two pieces of whole wheat bread in the afternoons, not realizing they were exacerbating his blood sugar woes. Meanwhile, things were going from bad to worse. His eye doctor, without knowing Eric had high blood sugar, told him he needed to do something about his blood sugar when he noticed ruptures in the tiny blood vessels in his eyes. Also, Eric was having constant pain in his feet, making it difficult for him to get to sleep at night.

Turning Point

That Christmas Eric's mother came for a visit, and when she and Deborah were out shopping, they came home and dropped a book in Eric's lap. They had discovered my book *60 Ways to Lower Your Blood Sugar* on a rack at the grocery store. Eric was intrigued and devoured the book. Hope sprang up immediately. He decided he had little to lose and became such a convert to the low-carb lifestyle that he made instant and drastic changes to his diet, far more than I have ever done. He went through his kitchen and threw out all the pasta, rice, and bread he could find.

I was intrigued. It was hard to imagine someone reading a single book and making such draconian changes so quickly. I asked him what it was about the book that moved him so deeply. He told me it was two things: first, my own experiences that I related in the book, and second, the simple thought that this would not be very difficult to try. If it didn't work, he could always go back to the way he had been eating before. After all, I wasn't advocating walking on hot coals or eating sharp nails. I was simply emphasizing a truth that nearly anyone who bothers to test their blood sugar could easily see: Lots of carbs raise blood sugar a lot, and few carbs raise it only a little. Eric decided he'd go from lots of carbs to fewer carbs and see what happened.

Before reading the book and reducing his carbs, his fasting blood sugar was often in the 140s. And of course, after eating his high-carb meals his blood sugar soared much higher. But now, with his determination to slash his carbs, his fasting blood sugar began to drop. After just one week, the fasting blood sugar was significantly lower. After two weeks, Eric noticed something he had not counted on—he started losing weight. By the time of the interview (less than one year after he started reducing his carbs) his weight had dropped from 235 to 190 without him making any conscious effort to lose weight! Eric had been far more concerned with blood sugar than weight loss. Since then I have received letters from him and his wife, and his weight had dropped more still.

Six months after Eric's previous visit to the doctor (when she had told him he would have to go on insulin if his A1C rose by one tenth of a point) he went to see her again. The difference was like day and night. His A1C had been 6.9. It was now 4.2. His triglycerides had been slashed from 347 to 158! His doctor was astonished. She asked what anybody would: "What on earth are you doing?" She told him she had never seen anyone experience such a huge change in so short a period of time and encouraged him, "Don't stop. Whatever it is you are doing, keep doing it!"

When I asked Eric about the specific factors that had helped him reduce carbs, he stated, "We read labels now, carefully. It's astonishing—the things in the grocery store that you pick up, read the label, and go: 'Holy cow, this is supposed to be good for you!'" He began checking on some of the recipes in his diabetic cookbooks and found that many of the recipes were high in carbs. Today he watches his carbs carefully and has normal blood sugar levels. He does allow himself desserts, but his go-to dessert these days is sugar-free Jell-O with strawberries.

Simple but Powerful

Eric Cooper represents many other people who have discovered the key to achieving normal blood sugar. I have lost count a long time ago of the many email testimonies I have received from people whose blood sugar levels have dropped to normal after reading my books and cutting their carbs. Eric has lost weight, his blood sugar is normal, and he is healthier now than he was years ago. He is not some freak exception who just happened to benefit from carbohydrate restriction. He is simply one more individual who found a powerful truth about overcoming runaway blood sugar: Slash the carbs, and your blood sugar begins to drop. It's not at all complicated. Best of all, it works for everybody: old people and young people, black people and white people, tall people and short people, extroverts and introverts, Baptists, Presbyterians, Pentecostals, and Buddhists. And it will work for you!

4

Breakfast: Getting a Good Start

No boxer would ever want to get knocked out in the first round. Of course, none would want to lose at all, but if you have to lose, you surely wouldn't want to make such a poor showing that you were beaten before you ever really began. Yet many diabetics beat themselves in the battle against high blood sugar by eating breakfasts that send their glucose levels soaring. For the rest of the day they are vainly trying to play catch-up. In this chapter we'll talk about meals and ways you can get off to a good start on your days, metabolically. But before we get into that, I need to share a couple of simple truths that serve as a foundation for the way I have attacked the monster of diabetes.

By this point you should be able to see that my approach to lowering blood sugar is an entirely pragmatic one. One definition of *pragmatic* is "dealing with things sensibly and realistically in a way that is based on practical rather than theoretical considerations."[1] In the realm of diabetes, theories abound. Many doctors, researchers, and authors begin their studies and writings with a built-in bias that colors all their views. I have no such bias. My approach is pretty simple. If something works to keep my blood sugar in the normal range, I will move in that direction. If a particular food or meal actually raises blood sugar, I will avoid it.

Considering the enormous danger that high blood sugar levels represent, the diabetic's greatest need is to get those blood sugar levels down in a hurry before they can do permanent damage to his or her body. If standing on your head an hour a day would significantly lower your blood sugar, you ought to be standing on your head daily. If dying your hair orange would do it, then you should run to the store and buy some orange hair dye without delay. But, of course, those things will do nothing to lower blood sugar. What will do it, without question, is to reduce the number of carbs you are eating daily and at every meal. Your blood sugar monitor will verify this again and again. You will easily see that nothing raises blood sugar like carbohydrates.

As you eat and test and eat and test some more, you will discover something that is quite liberating. You can make your blood sugar whatever you want it to be. I can get my blood sugar over 200, no problem. But I can also choose meals that barely budge my blood sugar, leaving it below 120 when it peaks an hour or so after I eat. So why should I choose a high-carb, high-starch, high-sugar meal that I know is going to send my blood sugar to the races when I could choose other foods that will have a minimal impact on blood sugar? The obvious answer is, I shouldn't.

Missing the Point

There are a great many so-called experts and nutritionists who have somehow missed this very basic point. I get a diabetic tip every week in my in-box from my health insurance carrier. Many of the tips are reasonable and could be helpful to diabetics. But one of them was just plain stupid. It said, "Use whole wheat pasta and low-fat cheese in your mac and cheese to add fiber and lower fat." They are saying it's okay to eat mac and cheese; just make sure the pasta is whole wheat and the cheese is low fat, and all will be fine. This is absolute nonsense. First, in many cases low fat does more harm than good for a diabetic when extra sugar is added, as explained previously. And second, what in the world would a diabetic be doing eating mac and cheese? This is just a small example of the uninformed and dangerous argument that says that diabetics merely have to change from white grain products to whole wheat and all their problems will be solved.

The one thing we desperately need to understand is that continual high blood sugar will gradually destroy our bodies, our organs, our eyesight, and our feet and legs. You've heard people say flippantly, "You're killing me!" That is exactly what high blood sugar (and its invisible cousin, high insulin) is doing to you, but it is doing it ever so quietly, one day at a time, over the course of months and years. A single high-carb meal is not that much of a problem. But when high carb—which is at the heart of the standard American diet, with all our breads, potatoes, sodas, sugar-filled desserts, fruit juices, doughnuts, and the like—becomes your lifestyle, you will eventually pay a terrible price for the "freedom" to eat whatever you like, as much as you like. It's not really a matter of if, but when.

I stated this in a previous book, but I think it bears repeating here. When you cut your carbs and take a pass on sugary desserts and the constant gorging on breads and pastries, you are not really going on a low-carb diet. You are simply eating the way the human race has eaten for most of the history of our world. It is the rest of America that is out of step. Instead of calling the lifestyle low carb, we might be more accurate to call it normal carb or reasonable carb. (Of course, that may sound kind of strange to others.)

When Our Blood Sugars Are Lowest

Enough preaching…let's talk about breakfast. When we wake up in the morning, in most cases our blood sugar is at its lowest point. If we haven't had a midnight snack, we've probably gone at least 8 and sometimes nearly 12 hours without eating. Full-fledged diabetics may already have glucose levels that are harmful, with fasting blood sugar in the 140s, 150s, and beyond. But many type 2 diabetics and prediabetics will find their fasting blood sugar between 100 and 110. At this point their blood sugar levels are not harming them. And it would be simple to keep those blood sugar levels down: Just don't eat anything all day long!

This is a major difference between a diabetic and an alcoholic. While the alcoholic can swear off the substance that is destroying him or her and never touch it again, the diabetic cannot simply abstain from food. To live we must eat. And it is food (and sugary drinks) that raise blood sugar. Water does not. Since we cannot simply give up food, cold-turkey or otherwise, we must be a little more discerning. One thing we *can* do is to give up certain types and classes of foods. We cannot say, "I will never eat again," but we can say, "I will never eat baked potatoes and chocolate cake again."

Another solution that would keep blood sugar low would be to simply eat meat and meat alone throughout the day: a big sirloin steak for breakfast, two grilled chicken breasts for lunch, and a large turkey drumstick for supper. These meals would barely nudge our blood sugar upward, and we would have great glucose control all day long. But we would be sadly lacking in the nutrients we need for optimum health, we would probably end up constipated, and we would find such a diet boring.

Meal Collecting

What we need is an arsenal of breakfast meals that raise our blood sugar gently and only slightly, and that will keep our numbers excellent right up until lunch. Our goal for breakfast (and every meal) is three-fold. First, we want to be able to become full or nearly so at each meal. If we cut our food intake so drastically that we are constantly hungry, we will never make it over the long haul. Second, we want meals that include a variety of vitamins and minerals. And third, it will be important that we find meals we actually enjoy. God created us with taste buds and made the ingestion of food to be pleasurable. To choose only foods that are low carb but taste like cardboard would decrease our motivation to stay the course.

The good news is that there are plenty of meals and plenty of breakfasts you can eat that should be perfectly fine for you—and that taste great! You just have to do a little reading, a little research, and be a tiny bit creative. Or if you are not creative, cruise the internet and do some low-carb searches.

Breakfast is important. It's the first meal of your day, and it's the key to setting the tone for a great day or a miserable day in terms of blood sugar. If possible, go for a walk or work out on a treadmill or an elliptical trainer before you sit down to eat your breakfast. But if you don't have time for that, realize that your body is still in a sluggish mode and probably not at its best to deal with blood sugar. Some of my highest blood sugar numbers have been when I have eaten a high-carb meal just after waking up from a nap or from a night's sleep. So go easy on your pancreas and give your body a light load at breakfast. To get up in the morning while your body is still working sluggishly and then down a couple of sweet rolls and a large glass of orange juice will create a blood sugar nightmare for a diabetic.

This brings us to the worst type of breakfast: What we call the "continental breakfast." The idea of a continental breakfast has come to us from Europe—and they should have kept it there! It normally contains foods that can be eaten quickly. And that means we're talking about sweet rolls and bagels and fruit and cereal and doughnuts and muffins… But what we are really talking about is carbs, carbs, and more carbs (and nearly all of them refined and processed).

I've been in motels that served only continental breakfasts. And when I saw what was being offered I turned around and went back to my room. I either ate a low-carb snack I had brought with me or went out to a restaurant for breakfast. A while back my wife and I stayed at a motel that provided a free breakfast. The problem was that nearly all it had to offer were high-carb, continental-type foods that were totally unacceptable and would drive my blood sugar crazy. However, amid the waffles, sweet rolls, fruit, toast, bagels, sugary yogurt, and fruit juice was a low-carb oasis. They had one small area where they provided scrambled eggs and sausage. Suddenly all was well. I might not get totally full, but at least I could get some low-carb food inside me, have a cup of coffee, and be about my day.

The Evil Doughnut

One American breakfast favorite that spells doom and gloom for diabetics and even nondiabetics is the doughnut. Doughnuts are one of the worst foods ever created. In all their different versions they contain almost no vitamins or nutrients. They are primarily a concoction of white flour and sugar. There is no room for compromise with doughnuts. Diabetics, prediabetics, and really everybody who draws breath on planet Earth should permanently swear off these things (I won't dignify them by calling them foods).

I went to a doughnut shop to film a piece about proper doughnut management. I demonstrated the one way to keep doughnuts from raising your blood sugar. You place the doughnut carefully on a napkin, wrap the napkin around the doughnut, squeeze the doughnut in the napkin, and then throw it into the trash.

While I was there I tested my 29-year-old cameraman, Jordan, after he ate two doughnuts, and what I discovered surprised even me.

Doughnut Test

While we were at the doughnut shop, I asked my 29-year-old cameraman if he would like to test himself with the doughnut. He is not a diabetic, and his pre-test revealed a great glucose number of 73 mg/dl. One hour after eating two doughnuts his blood sugar soared to 183. If a nondiabetic young man in his twenties can see a blood sugar rise of 110 points in about an hour after two doughnuts, what do you suppose would happen to a full-fledged diabetic? The moral of the story: Doughnuts and other sweet pastries are not your friend. The flour alone in the pastry will raise blood sugar, but with all the sugar they put on top and within, the doughnut is an absolute monster when it comes to blood sugar control.

DOUGHNUT TEST (JORDAN —29 YEARS OLD)	
	2 Doughnuts
Before Eating	73
After 1 Hour	183
Total Blood sugar Rise	110 mg/dl

Summary: These results were a surprise to both of us! Here was a young man whose blood sugar processing ought to be outstanding, and yet he was having a problem dealing with the starch and sugar from two doughnuts. The glucose peak of 183 was way too high. A 110-point blood sugar rise in an hour is unhealthy and abnormal. Jordan is surely representative of people everywhere who eat doughnuts regularly and never even consider what they may be doing to their blood sugar levels and their health.

Unnatural Fruit Juice

While we are on the subject of terrible breakfast fare, let me give dishonorable mention to what is considered a breakfast staple for many Americans: fruit juice. For some reason many folks feel like breakfast just isn't complete if they don't have a good-sized glass of orange juice, grape juice, or apple juice. And if you question them about it, they will reply indignantly, "This juice has fruit in it, so it must be natural and has to be good for you!"

They are exactly wrong! Fruit juice is so highly concentrated that the megadoses of sugar you are getting from the juice is totally unnatural. Overwhelming your body with sugar is not what the Creator of fruit ever intended. If you're going to eat fruit with your breakfast, eat a whole orange, or better yet, half an orange (or a whole mandarin). Whole fruit is not without its problems for diabetics, but it's far superior to fruit juice due to its fiber content and the fact that its sugar is not nearly so concentrated. Stay away from that sugar-laden concoction we know as fruit juice, whether grape juice, pineapple juice, orange juice, or mango juice. Eating a single fruit can be problematic for many diabetics. Drinking fruit juice is simply disastrous.

One of the problems with breakfast is that many Americans are in such a rush in the mornings that they are unable (or unwilling) to take the time to make and eat a hot meal. And many of the foods that are quick are usually high in carbs. Toaster pastries are a good example of this. You don't have to fry a toaster pastry. You don't have to cook a toaster pastry. You just put it in the toaster and in about a minute, pop goes the toaster, and your sugary, starchy, unhealthy toaster pastry is ready, with its nearly 40 grams of carbs. If you eat two, the way many people do, you're up to between 70 and 80 grams. Add a glass of orange juice and you're over 100!

Grape Juice vs. Coca-Cola Test

Some foods for the diabetic are obviously dangerous. When you find out that you have a problem with processing carbs and sugars, you say to yourself, "All right, I'd better go easy on desserts and lay off soda." Sadly, not every diabetic even goes this far. Some just go right on eating and drinking exactly as they did before, thinking perhaps they'll be one of the lucky ones who never suffer diabetic complications, which is highly unlikely.

As I said before, it seems that many people feel breakfast just is not complete without a glass of fruit juice. What better way to get your morning off to a good start than with all those vitamins? After all, fruit juice is made from fruit, and it is so…natural! Soda is bad, fruit juice is good; soda is unnatural, fruit juice is natural; soda is man-made, fruit juice is nature-made.

As I love to do, I decided to do a blood sugar test contrasting the blood sugar–raising properties of Coca-Cola versus Welch's Grape Juice. (It was, in fact, Welch's Black Cherry Concord Grape Juice, which is made up of four different fruit juices, with grape juice being predominant.) When I was a boy, my mom used to buy good old Welch's Grape Juice, and I loved it. But as an adult and a prediabetic, how would it affect my blood sugar? Before doing the test, I knew one thing: Both the soda and the grape juice would produce a fairly significant blood sugar rise. But would the man-made Coca-Cola be much worse than the "natural" grape juice? I did not have to wonder or theorize about this. My blood sugar monitor would give me the definitive answer. My guess was that they would be pretty close in their blood sugar–raising properties.

Soda vs. Grape Juice Test

For each test I poured the drinks into a measuring cup until they reached the 12-ounce mark. I would be getting exactly the same amount of soda or juice each time. For the first test I drank the Coca-Cola. I decided to do a 30-minute post-test, along with a one-hour post-test. I had not drunk a Coke in years, and I have to admit, it tasted pretty good. The Coke raised my blood sugar from 99 to 149 at 30 minutes, but by the one hour mark it was already going back down. At one hour my monitor read 139. My pancreas was obviously working hard, dumping out insulin to deal with all that sugar. At its peak, the Coke raised my blood sugar 50 points. How would it compare with the grape juice?

One day later I poured out 12 ounces of grape juice into a measuring cup and drank it. When I do these blood sugar tests, I am sometimes surprised at the results, and this was one of those times. It turned out that the grape juice raised my blood sugar higher than the soda, both at the 30-minute mark and the one-hour mark. After 30 minutes, the grape juice had raised my blood sugar from 103 to 196. Wow! That's a huge rise—93 points in a half hour. As with the Coke, by an hour it was already back on its way down. The one-hour post-test read was 173. Sugary drinks, when taken by themselves on an empty stomach, hit your system fast. They raise blood sugar rapidly, and afterward it tends to start dropping rapidly as well. To my surprise, Welch's Grape Juice was the "winner" in this contest—but winning the "raise your blood sugar the highest" trophy is a pretty dubious honor!

SODA VS. GRAPE JUICE TEST		
	Coca-Cola	Welch's Grape Juice
Before Eating	99	103
After 30 Minutes	149	196
After 1 Hour	139	173
Total Blood sugar Rise	50 mg/dl	93 mg/dl

Summary: Here is proof once more that just because a product is related to or is fruit, it is not good for diabetics. The grape juice was a nightmare for my blood sugar. And remember, almost no one drinks fruit juice alone. They usually have it with a snack or a meal. And if that meal contains a significant amount of carbs, the grape juice will just add to all the other sugary and starchy foods to produce a total glucose disaster. And if a prediabetic like me can see a nearly 100-point rise in blood sugar, what would happen to a true diabetic?

One more word about the grape juice: there is something terribly ironic about the way Welch's markets this product. They tout their grape juice as about the healthiest thing you could possibly drink. On their label they proudly declare that it is "100% juice." They boast about how there is no sugar added. And they announce that you get two servings of fruit when you guzzle this sugar-laden, blood sugar–raising juice. In truth, there was no need for them to add sugar. They have concentrated this product to such a degree that it is overloaded with natural sugar. And gullible Americans and even diabetics drink it, naively assuming that they are doing their body a favor.

Proper Breakfasts

In America we have definite assumptions and traditions about what a proper breakfast ought to be. We have looked at some of the bad traditions, which include doughnuts, most cereals, bagels, toaster pastries, and so forth. But some of our traditional foods are no problem whatsoever for blood sugar. The classic breakfast of eggs and bacon is a great example. Eggs and bacon have almost no carbs. An egg has about .4 grams of carbs, so you can eat three eggs and you'll get about one gram of carbs—basically nothing. Bacon has even less—about one-tenth of one gram of carbs per bacon slice. So you'd have to eat ten slices of bacon to work your way up to one gram of carbs! What this means is that, unless you are a type 1 diabetic, eggs and bacon will have virtually no impact on your blood sugar.

Now, if you have bought into the idea that the ideal diet is low fat and eating foods with almost no cholesterol, you'll probably be scared to death of a bacon-and-eggs breakfast. But many researchers and nutritionists are now saying that low-fat diets actually improve your likelihood of obesity and diabetes due to their potency of provoking a high degree of insulin release.[2] When American nutritionists and the federal government officially sanctioned the low-fat, high-carb diet, America's health took a decided turn for the worse.[3] And when Robert Atkins had the audacity to write a book in the '70s about the benefits of low-carb, high-fat eating, he was labeled a heretic. But the problem was, as more Americans began losing weight on his diet, the researchers converged on this diet, determined to prove that although you might lose weight, you would surely drop over dead of a heart attack and never make it past your forties. Then a strange thing happened. The test results and studies showed that not only did people lose weight on a low-carb diet, but they also saw tremendous results in their blood sugar levels—and their triglycerides (a measure of fat in the blood) plummeted.[4]

Slowly (very slowly) the federal government has admitted they were a bit overzealous and has changed their dietary guidelines. They have declared that eggs, for example, are safe to eat after all, reversing their views after 40 years of telling us that eggs are terrible for us.[5] Think of all those unfortunate souls who faithfully discarded their egg yolks and ate only the white part now finding out that their sacrifice was for nothing! Of course, no one wants to eat eggs and bacon every morning. But as you read and research, you will discover that there are all kinds of wonderful breakfasts that will keep your blood sugar safe and humming along at reasonable levels.

Fruit on the Breakfast Table

One of our American traditions is to have fruit on our breakfast tables every morning. You may be able to enjoy fruit for breakfast, but you have to be careful, and you absolutely cannot have as much fruit and as many different kinds of fruit as you would probably like. Strawberries are a great fruit for diabetics. A small to medium strawberry has only one gram of carbs. If your main breakfast food is fairly low-carb, you can add several strawberries and still be just fine. Melons are a bit lower in carbs than other fruits, so you may be able add small portions of melons to relatively low-carb breakfasts, but you will have to be careful. They are not all that low-carb!

Fruit is tasty and filled with vitamins and nutrients, so whenever you can add small amounts of fruit to a meal and still keep it under your maximum limit, do so. But don't allow fruit to become so paramount to you that you eat it at the cost of safe blood sugar levels! When you have apples, oranges, or bananas (if your body can tolerate them), eat half at a time, and then test an hour later. If you can get away with it, great. If not, say adios to fruit and go with foods that are lower in carbs.

Low-Carb Pancakes

I discovered low-carb pancakes after discovering I was prediabetic and insulin resistant. I have always loved routines. I suppose it has something to do with feeling secure by making my life as predictable as possible. One of my routines that has endured nearly all my adult life is the practice of sitting down to a Saturday morning breakfast of pancakes and sausage. Pancakes require a little more time and effort to make than most other breakfasts, and so Saturday seems the ideal day for them. In my pre-blood sugar–problems days, I had pancakes the old-fashioned way, made from a mix that came in a box and liberally drenched with pancake syrup. I never thought about it, but the meal I was enjoying so much was a blood sugar disaster. Even as a young adult I can remember feeling jittery around lunchtime, after all those pancakes with syrup no doubt caused a rapid blood sugar rise, which led to an insulin dump, which then caused an even more rapid blood sugar drop. In those days I never thought about such things and simply wondered why I felt so strange on Saturdays.

When I gained a little knowledge about the carbohydrate-and-blood sugar-rise connection and my own insulin resistance, I knew I had to make some changes. But giving up on Saturday morning pancakes was painful to even contemplate. I was pleased to quickly discover the blessing of using soy flour and heavy whipping cream to make an alternative version of the typical pancake. My post-test monitor readings were excellent. My blood sugar hardly rose at all. And the taste was nearly as nice as what I had given up. Saturday pancakes were back on the menu.

This was one of the earlier substitutions I discovered and employed, and I have stayed with it for many years, even to the present time. I do not consider this switch to a different version of pancakes a major sacrifice. In fact, it is hardly a sacrifice at all. I sometimes put a few mashed strawberries or blueberries on my pancakes and a little whipped cream. Anyone seeing me eat such a treat would surely think I had fallen off the low-carb wagon, but in truth I am riding right in the center of that wagon. When my blood sugar peaks in the low hundreds, I know I am doing just fine!

Pancake Test

I conducted three blood sugar tests to demonstrate the radical difference between eating pancakes the regular way: store-bought pancake mix with regular sugary pancake syrup and two versions of pancakes quite low in carbohydrates. One low-carb pancake was the soy pancakes mentioned above. And for good measure I tested myself after eating pancakes made primarily with coconut flour and eggs.

PANCAKE TEST			
	Regular Pancakes, Regular Syrup	Soy Flour Pancakes, Sugar-Free Syrup	Coconut Flour Pancakes, Sugar-Free Syrup
Before Eating	104	88	98
After 1 Hour	167	93	99
Total Blood sugar Rise	63 mg/dl	5 mg/dl	1 mg/dl

Summary: What a contrast this demonstrates! With the two, low-carb pancake meals my blood sugar rose 1 mg/dl and 5 mg/dl. But with the normal pancakes, and using regular pancake syrup, my blood sugar rose 63 mg/dl—and into the dangerous 167 range. Turns out I have been saving myself a lot of high blood sugar by eating low-carb pancakes with sugar-free syrup nearly every Saturday for the last 16 years!

Regular Pancakes/Sugar-Free Syrup

Afterward, I decided to test myself with the two regular pancakes, using sugar-free syrup, which should have a minimal effect on blood sugar.

The day after eating the two regular pancakes smothered with normal, sugary syrup, I ate two similar pancakes, but this time used sugar-free syrup. My blood sugar did not rise quite so high, but it still rose too much, peaking at the one-hour after-meal mark at 150.

PANCAKE TEST—REGULAR SYRUP VS. SUGAR-FREE SYRUP		
	2 Regular Pancakes, Regular Syrup	2 Regular Pancakes, Sugar-Free Syrup
Before Eating	104	94
After 1 Hour	167	150
Total Blood sugar Rise	63 mg/dl	56 mg/dl

Summary: These contrasting tests make an important point: even without the sugary syrup, the bread content of the pancakes produced a significant rise in blood sugar. Too often diabetics assume that if they eliminate sweet-tasting foods they have done enough. But as we see in tests like these, that is clearly not enough. Breads and starches are able to significantly raise blood sugar all by themselves.

There is one further consideration I need to mention about these tests that also applies to many other tests found in this book. The portions I had were moderate. In this case I was eating two medium-sized pancakes with two small sausages as my breakfast. My constant vigilance over my blood sugar levels has caused moderate portions to become normal for me. There was a time when I never would have been satisfied with two pancakes. In my younger years I would have eaten at least three and sometimes four. And this is precisely the way many Americans do eat. These numbers do not really reflect the way the average pancake breakfast would affect many Americans, especially the normal pancake/normal syrup breakfast. Many would eat more pancakes and see a significantly higher blood sugar rise if they had the same measure of insulin resistance that I have, or worse.

One other thought: Some folks have the habit of pouring pancake syrup over every individual pancake in their stack (rather than just the top), which multiplies the sugar and carbs two- or three- or fourfold— and their blood sugar levels, if they checked them, would scream out a warning to them to stop such an unhealthy practice. What a nightmare a pancake breakfast can be if one is not discriminating and does not make the needed substitutions!

A Week of Breakfasts

As I was putting together a video about breakfasts for diabetics, I decided to keep track of my own breakfast one-hour post-meal blood sugar peaks for an entire working week.

Breakfast Blood Sugar Peaks

On Monday through Friday of that week, I faithfully recorded my blood sugar numbers one hour after breakfast. I didn't bother to test myself before my meals since my morning fasting blood sugar is nearly always in the same general range. But each morning I set my timer for one hour after taking my last bite and sip of coffee. My meals were my go-to low-carb meals throughout these five days. Each day I saw good numbers, and after a week I was satisfied that I have been kind to my pancreas.

A WEEK OF 1-HOUR POST-BREAKFAST BLOOD SUGAR PEAKS		
	Breakfast	Blood sugar Peak
Monday	Eggs, Bacon, *Biscuit and Gravy	108
Tuesday	Low-Carb Pancakes with Sugar-Free Syrup, Sausage	100
Wednesday	3 Eggs with Sausage and Low-Carb Muffins	101
Thursday	Eggs, Bacon, and ½ Low-Carb Bagel with Cheese	108
Friday	Coconut Low-Carb Pancakes, Sausage, Sugar-Free Syrup	106

Summary: My average for these five days was 104 at the one-hour post-meal peak. I was happy with that. It feels great to see those kinds of numbers and to know that you have been kind and gentle to your body! And when we are kind to our bodies, they'll be kind to us!

*A biscuit with gravy can hardly qualify as low-carb. But sometimes I will take a regular biscuit, cut a section of the middle out, and eat the thin top and bottom. I find my body can normally handle this, although for many diabetics, it would be better to avoid this or substitute a low-carb biscuit.

Let me share with you a little secret: I fully expected to get good results like these. The reason I expected this was not because I don't have blood sugar problems, and it wasn't because I'm not insulin resistant, because I am. The reason I expected good results and good numbers was because I was eating meals that I had tested many times before, and I knew by experience that they would make little impact on my blood sugar. When you have done several tests on a particular meal and found that each time you eat it your blood sugar barely rises, it becomes like an old friend to you. You feel you can trust it, and that is a great feeling!

Being Bad on Saturday

Saturday was a different story. This day I deliberately set about to break my own rules and eat a more normal (SAD: Standard American Diet) breakfast.

Breaking the Rules

After five good days of breakfast blood sugar peaks, I headed for my local fast-food restaurant and ordered a breakfast that included a little bit of everything: eggs, sausage, two pancakes with syrup, hash browns, and a medium-sized glass of orange juice. From experience with all the blood sugar tests I have done over many years, I knew this breakfast was going to be different from the previous five. For the last five days my breakfast blood sugar peaks never even reached 110. This time it would be different.

After breakfast we did some shopping and went to a few garage sales. Knowing I would be driving around town, I brought two things with me that I would need: my timer and my blood sugar monitor. When my timer went off, I happened to be driving, so I simply pulled off the side of the road (don't do this on major highways!) and tested myself. Because I was doing this for a video I was making, my wife stepped outside the car and held the camera on me while I tested and talked. The monitor gave me a reading of 145, actually somewhat lower than I had anticipated, but still significantly higher than the 104 average peak I had experienced over the previous five days.

FIVE-DAY AVERAGE WITH LOW-CARB BREAKFASTS VS. HIGH-CARB FAST-FOOD BREAKFAST		
	5-Day Average with Low-Carb Breakfasts	Fast-Food High-Carb Breakfast
1-Hour Peak	104	145

Summary: I was surprised that the fast-food breakfast did not raise my blood sugar higher than it did, especially since I drank that super-sugary orange juice and covered my pancakes with that nasty (but sweet) syrup. Blood sugar tests do yield their surprises! Apparently our pancreases do better on some days than others. Also, the fat from the sausage probably kept the carbs from raising my blood sugar as high as it would have risen had I eaten pure carbs without any fat. Still, comparing the 104-average peak of the low-carb breakfasts with the 145 after fast-food breakfast, my basic expectation held true. My blood sugar did indeed rise significantly higher with high-carb than low-carb.

It's in Your Hands

As I contrast the Monday through Friday meals with the Saturday breakfast, there is some great news—something I stress in every book I write and emphasize in every video I produce on this subject. The news is this: what you put in your mouth makes a huge difference in the levels to which your blood sugar rises. This means that if you are like most type 2 diabetics, you are in control of how far your blood sugar is going to rise. The choices you make are going to give you either high blood sugar, moderately high blood sugar, or normal blood sugar. Change your diet and you can easily change your blood sugar levels. It is true that people with insulin resistance have less dietary choices than normal folks, if they want to keep their blood sugar in bounds. But it is also true that with a little research you can find that you have a whole lot more choices than you originally thought you did.

I like that! I like that I have quite a bit of control in this business. High blood sugar is not some uncontrollable, mysterious illness that is beyond any human intervention. It is, in fact, one of the most "controllable" diseases you could possibly have. Yes, it is a little frustrating that some people just process carbs and sugars much better than we do. When I ate that Saturday breakfast at the fast-food restaurant, my wife had nearly the same breakfast, but her blood sugar peaked at 106, a whole lot better than my 145. That doesn't seem fair! She did as well with a high-carb breakfast as I usually do with a low-carb breakfast. That's something I can't do much about, but I can adjust my own meals and diet so that my blood sugar doesn't go out of control and ends up pretty much matching my wife's. She just has the luxury of more meal choices than I do. But that's okay. I can live with that, knowing that I am saving myself a world of health issues by watching what I eat.

5

Nutrition for the Diabetic

Have you ever given much thought to the two food groups known as fruits and vegetables? If you are diabetic, you should! In this chapter, we are going to look at the idea of nutrition as it relates to diabetes. Jesus once remarked, "What will it profit a man if he gains the whole world, and loses his own soul?" (Mark 8:36). In the area of diabetes, we might ask, "What profit is it to a man or a woman if they get their blood sugar under control by cutting their carbs, losing weight, and exercising, but take in such poor nutrition and so few essential vitamins and nutrients that they become susceptible to a host of other afflictions and diseases?"

Our main goal in dealing with runaway blood sugar is not simply to get our blood sugar numbers lower and leave it at that. Our goal should be good health—period! And that will involve nutrition.

The goal is to find nutritious foods to eat that will not send our blood sugar into the stratosphere. I can't just live on meat, of course, but there are lots of great, low-carb vegetables that pass the test as well. And there are some fruits that aren't too bad in smaller portions. There are even certain types of bread that can be handled easily. But you have to find these and sort out the good from the bad. This means you have to test, test, test yourself, and read, research, and watch videos on the low-carb lifestyle. In time you will discover what your body can tolerate, and you can begin shaping a lifestyle and an eating pattern that will work for you.

Food and Nutrients

There was once a time when people did not realize that food contained various vitamins, minerals, and nutrients. The only thing they knew was that when you ate food you lost your hunger, and when you skipped food you got hungry, you got skinny, and you eventually died. So putting two and two together, people concluded that food is good for you. And they were right! Food is good for you, but some food is a whole lot better for you than others, and there are some foods that will make you much healthier if you throw them in the trash rather than eating them. We call things that belong in the trash garbage, which is precisely what some "foods" are. Pretzels, chips, doughnuts, sugary desserts, and sodas are far healthier for you when thrown in your trash can than when put them into your stomach, where they will force your pancreas to go into emergency mode and pump its little guts out while your body become progressively more insulin resistant and you eat yourself into an early grave.

When we think about healthy foods, we normally think about fruits and vegetables. In fact, this connection is made so often they are typically and unbreakably linked together in the minds of many: fruits… and vegetables. We're told that if you want to be healthy, eat lots of fruits and vegetables. But for diabetics and the prediabetics, fruits and vegetable are not created equal. In truth, fruits are far more problematic for those who struggle with blood sugar problems than most vegetables. It is important that I use the qualifying word *most* because there are some vegetables, such as potatoes and corn, that are loaded with starches and will convert to sugar in your bodies with blazing speed. If you avoid the sweet-tasting fruits but load up on potatoes, you are doing yourself no favor!

Fruit Superior to Candy

There are two major reasons why fruit is superior to candy, pies, cakes, and so forth. First, at least with the fruit you are getting nutrition as a consolation for the sweet sugar you are ingesting. There is no vitamin C in chocolate cake, soda, or a candy bar, but you get twice your daily requirement in a full-sized orange. So while the sugar may be a little tough on your pancreas, the nutrients are doing your body a favor.

Second, the sugar you get in fruit is not on its own. It is typically locked up in fiber, which means that it will take longer to hit your blood stream, and the extra time it takes for your body to process it helps reduce blood sugar spikes. Your blood sugar will surely rise, but it won't rise quite so high as it will with foods lacking fiber. Typically ingesting a large banana will not result in a blood sugar peak as high was one you would get when eating a piece of cake with the same amount of carbs. The 50 grams of carbs in a mango will probably not give you as high a post-meal blood sugar peak as drinking 18 ounces of soda will.

What this means is that if you have to choose between an orange and a candy bar, by all means go for the orange. If some man breaks in your house with a gun, and forces you at gunpoint to either eat a banana or drink a soda, choose the banana for sure! But since we are unlikely to be forced to choose, it would make sense for us to be a little hesitant to eat a lot of fruit when we eat get healthy, nutritious vegetables instead and be a whole lot kinder to our pancreases.

Bananas vs. Candy Bars Test

In thinking about the differences between fruit and candy, I finally decided to put the two to the test and discover just how much advantage fruit is over candy, when the carbohydrate count is nearly the same for the two. I decided to compare bananas with Hershey's chocolate bars. Large bananas have around 30 grams of carbs and the chocolate bars have 28. So I chose a couple of bananas that seemed bigger than medium but not quite large. I figured that these bananas should be right around 28 grams of carbs. I was curious just what kind of a difference I would find in terms of their blood sugar–raising capacity.

I decided to do this experiment on two consecutive days. On the first day I would eat two bananas for my breakfast, and on the second day I would have the two Hershey's chocolate bars. In each case I tested myself one hour after finishing my "meal." I have to admit, the results surprised me. I was almost certain that the candy bars would raise my blood sugar higher than the bananas, but it didn't prove to be the case. After the two tests I obtained these results:

Before my banana meal, my blood sugar was at 106. After 30 minutes it had risen to 192. And one hour after eating the bananas it rose still higher—to 222. I knew the bananas would raise my blood sugar significantly, but I didn't know they would raise it that high! The next day was my Hershey's bar breakfast. Before the meal, my blood sugar was once again at 106. Thirty minutes after finishing the candy bars, it had risen to 151, my first clue that the candy was affecting my blood sugar less than the bananas. And at the one-hour mark, my blood sugar rose to 169. With the bananas there was a 116-point rise, and with the candy bars there was a 63-point rise.

BANANAS VS. CANDY BAR TEST		
	2 Bananas	2 Hershey's Bars
Before Eating	106	106
After 30 Minutes	192	151
After 1 Hour	222	169
Total Blood sugar Rise	116 mg/dl	63 mg/dl

Summary: This was a shocker! I fully expected that the candy bars would raise my blood sugar higher than the bananas. As it turned out, the bananas not only raised it higher, but significantly higher. The candy bars did have significant fat in them, which tends to moderate blood sugar spikes. This may explain why the bananas raised my blood sugar so much higher. But there is no getting around the fact that the bananas raised my blood sugar big-time. What is the moral of this story? It's not that candy is preferable! It demonstrates that for diabetics, fruit may not be quite as innocuous as you think. Be careful and eat fruit moderately.

Now, in order to make this a truly scientific experiment I would have to repeat this test many times. And I was not about to do that. I had abused my body enough with these two high-carb breakfasts as it was, and I was eager to get back to my traditional low-carb breakfasts. Still, there are some things we can learn. First, I learned that for me, bananas are a real problem when it comes to raising blood sugar. I already knew that, but it was driven home far more forcefully after these two tests. Remember, however, we are all different in regard to our ability to process sugars and carbs. The results may not be at all the same for you. But for me, and I would think for most diabetics, bananas are problematic, to say the least. And that goes for most fruit. Berries are relatively safe, and eating half pieces of fruit can be made to work with certain meals, but we need to be prudent.

The truth is, fruit does not get a free pass just because it contains more vitamins and nutrients than many other foods. What profit is it to a man or a woman to get that extra calcium in bananas while they drive their blood sugar crazy and damage their bodies. There is some wonderful encouragement in this little experiment. It is the same thing I have been saying in my books and in nearly every diabetes video we produce. The encouraging truth is this: *We can make a difference in how high our blood sugar rises.* We are not helpless victims who have no say in the matter. Nobody forced me to eat those two bananas or those two candy bars. I chose to do it, and the consequences were runaway blood sugar. But what if instead I had eaten two avocados or two celery stalks filled with cream cheese? Do you suppose I would have seen better numbers? You better believe I would!

Your Amazing Pancreas

Let's talk about the pancreas for a moment. The key organ that regulates blood sugar in our bodies is our pancreas. The pancreas is truly miraculous. It was designed to process blood sugars in our bodies regardless of how much or how little sugar we throw at it. Whether we eat candy, cakes, and pies loaded with processed sugar, or we eat pasta, potatoes, rice, bread, and other starchy foods that are rapidly converted to sugar, our pancreas is normally ready and able to handle it all. It was made by our Creator to last us a lifetime—70, 80, 90 years—and for many people it does just that.

But when we abuse our pancreas by overdosing on sugars, refined, processed carbs, starches, pasta, bread, doughnuts, bagels, and the like, we can eventually blow it out until it barely functions. In addition to our blatant disregard for healthy eating, our lack of exercise, being overweight, and living continually with high insulin levels can lead us to become insulin resistant. (Very simply, it's when cells in the liver, body fat, and muscles resist insulin's important signal to let glucose pass from the blood into cells that need it for fuel. When this happens, glucose, or sugar, builds up in the blood stream, which causes the pancreas to crank out more insulin.) And the older we get, the more likely we are to struggle with processing blood sugar. Typically, the more insulin resistant we are, the harder we work our pancreas, and the harder we work it, the more inefficient we become metabolically. We end up living with five, ten, or twenty times as much insulin in our bloodstream as is normal. And this leads to still more insulin resistance, which forces our overworked pancreas to dump still more insulin, which creates more insulin resistance, and…well, I think you get the idea! You can see where all this will end: raging diabetes for those who are genetically inclined in that direction. They may then experience all kinds of physical complications, such as foot pain and the loss of our eyesight, and in the end, premature death. It is not a pretty picture, and millions have gone this way, completely clueless that they were gradually destroying their body, bite by high-carb bite, meal by meal, and day by day. (Some people can get away with high-sugar, high-carb diets and a lack of exercise, and still not become diabetic. But because you are reading this book, chances are you are not one of them.)

Car Abuse and Body Abuse

Let's think about a new car. When you purchase a new car, you expect that it will last you many years. Unless you are wealthy and can afford to change your car every three years, you may feel that you should be able to get ten good years out of a new car, at the very least. But what if the various components of this car begin to fail after only a year and a half? You would feel cheated. Let's imagine a man who goes into his car dealership to complain about the vehicle he purchased less than two years ago. The manager asks him a few questions about the car, and the man admits that at one point he drained the oil out of his car to give it to his poor cousin, Billy Bob, and never bothered to replace it.

The manager is astonished, asking the irate customer, "You mean you have been driving your car around without oil since then?" The man shakes his head sadly and laments, "Well, actually, after I drained out all the oil, that car only lasted me a couple of days. After that the engine overheated and seized up, and it hasn't run since. I've tinkered around with it a little bit, but nothing works. The car acts as though it will never run again." The manager tells the man in no uncertain terms that he has totally abused his car and that he has no one to blame but himself. He was operating that vehicle in a manner it was never intended. And just as no car can run without oil, neither can we humans drive our vehicles (our bodies) through this life and expect them to give us long and faithful service while we constantly abuse them by stuffing our mouths with refined, processed carbs and sugars, and more carbs and more sugars, morning, noon, and night.

Fruits and Veggies

Getting back to fruits and vegetables, sometimes you hear the expression "The most bang for your buck." This is precisely the idea behind focusing heavily on vegetables and lightly on fruits. Both fruits *and* vegetables are loaded with vitamins and nutrients. But vegetables (most of them) give you the most nutrition for the carbs they possess, the most bang for your buck. If I can get loads of vitamins and nutrients by eating a salad, which will hardly affect my blood sugar, and I can also get lots of vitamins and nutrients by eating fruits, which will seriously raise my blood sugar, which should I choose: the fruit or the salad? Well, that's a no-brainer. Both may give you nutrition, but one gives you nutrition without too many carbs and the other gives you nutrition along with a whole lot of carbs and natural sugars.

The idea is to lean toward the vegetables and cut back on the fruit. I know what some of you are saying: "But fruit is so natural; it must be good for you." In truth the fruit you buy at your grocery store is not all that natural. Most of the fruit you see in the produce department has been genetically modified and altered through cross-breeding until it possesses far more sugar than fruit your great-great-grandfather ate. And remember this: Your great-great-grandpa typically only ate fruit in season. A couple of months after the fruit ripened and was picked, it was either eaten or it was rotten. And grandpa was done with fruit for nearly a year, until the next harvest came along. But today we can run to our grocery store, winter, spring, summer, or fall, fill our shopping carts with fruit, and satisfy our sugar cravings any time we like.

All this being said, as I have mentioned, it is not necessary to give up on fruit altogether. I still eat fruit, but in moderation. I eat apples, but usually only a half an apple at a time, and only when I am eating a meal that is otherwise quite low in carbs. I normally don't eat regular oranges, but I eat the little mini version called clementines. As with nearly all that I eat, I found out by testing myself that I can get away with it when I allow myself a clementine in certain specific situations. In order to make this point I did the following test.

Clementine Test

Typically, when you begin to really see what an unbreakable link there is between carbs and high blood sugar, your life and your diet change in a hurry! At first you are far more aware of what you cannot or should not eat than what you *can* eat. Large numbers of foods and snacks are ripped out of your life. And because you will almost immediately see a tremendous improvement in your blood sugar numbers, fasting blood sugar, and A1C scores, you will hopefully become quite serious and conscientious about the amount of carbs you allow yourself per day and per meal.

This certainly was the case for me. And in my zeal to get good numbers, I sometimes wiped out entire categories of foods without discrimination. Fruit is a perfect example. When I became convinced that natural sugar can significantly raise blood sugar, I was done with fruit. Good-bye apples, so long oranges, sayonara pineapples! But once my blood sugar was brought under control, and I lost my early fanaticism about completely wiping carbs from my diet and my vocabulary, I took another look at it. The reason was not that I love fruit so much that I couldn't stand to give it up. It was rather that fruit is so bursting with vitamins and nutrients that if there was a way to eat limited portions in a controlled manner, it seemed wise and right that I should take a second look at fruit.

One example of a fruit that works for me is the clementine. These sweet little treats go by the brand names Cuties and Halos in most stores. They are probably less than half the size, calories, and carbs of a normal orange, but they are just about as sweet, and more importantly, they provide over 100 percent of our daily requirement for vitamin C. There are different estimates for the carbohydrates found in these mini oranges, sometimes also called mandarins, but one source lists them as having 9 grams of carbs, with 1 gram of fiber. This would equal 8 net grams of carbs (carbs that actually affect blood sugar). As I thought about this—100 percent of vitamin C for only 8 grams of carbs—I realized that this fits into the "lots of bang for the buck" category.

I wasn't about to allow these extra 8 grams to push me over the edge of the 140 mg/dl peak limit I have set for myself, but I was pretty sure that with some of my lower-carb meals, I could probably squeeze one of these bad boys in without going past the boundary. I thought about a low-carb breakfast I usually enjoy around once a week. This meal involves one-half of a light English muffin, an egg, sausage, and cheese. I normally leave off the top part of the muffin. Because the muffin, being a *light* muffin, has 17 grams of carbs total, and I am only using half of it, I am only getting around 9 grams of carbs for the bread. The cheese, sausage, and egg are quite minimal and might add perhaps 3 more grams of carbs. This "Dennis McMuffin" has only around 12 grams of carbs. And I know by experience that I can usually handle most breakfast meals and keep my blood sugar numbers in good shape as long as I stay at or under 25 grams of carbs. So I figured that adding 8 more grams by having a "Halo" to the 12 grams of the muffin should leave me in good shape.

Dennis McMuffin Plus Clementine

Wanting to do this experiment scientifically, I scheduled two different breakfasts on consecutive days: the first day I would eat only the muffin for breakfast, having had no food since the previous evening. The second morning, under the same conditions, I would eat a similar muffin plus one Halo mandarin orange. Having tested myself countless times with various foods and carb counts, I wasn't expecting either meal to seriously raise my blood sugar. And I was correct.

After eating the sausage, cheese, and egg muffin (no top), my blood sugar rose from 102 before the meal to 107 one hour after the meal, a five-point rise. Nothing wrong with that! Of course, I had only ingested around 12 grams of carbohydrate. Most type 2 diabetics should be able to eat this kind of a meal and keep their blood sugar in the safe range. Still, looking at the beautiful 107 on my monitor and knowing that I would not be eating anything else until lunch was a good feeling. My blood sugars were guaranteed to be in the safe range for a third of the day!

The next morning I was eager to see what the additional clementine would do to me. The sweetness of the little mini orange made the meal more pleasurable, and all that was left was to see if those 8 additional grams of carbs would result in a significantly higher blood sugar level. I didn't think they would, and I was right!

One hour after my meal of a "Dennis McMuffin" plus one Halo, my blood sugar was lower than it had been the day before. Before this meal my blood sugar was at 109. Clearly this was higher than doctors like our fasting blood sugar to be. Anyone with a morning blood sugar of 109 has definite diabetic tendencies and is headed for trouble if they do not watch their diet. But of course, I do watch my diet, and have been doing so for a long time.

Interestingly, my blood sugar test one hour after the meal read 99—a ten-point drop! Now, this may be a little bit puzzling for many. The previous day, with just the sausage muffin, it rose five points, whereas this day, with an additional 8 grams of carbs from the mini orange, it decreased by ten points. What's the deal? You may be thinking, *I thought the more carbs you eat, the higher your blood sugar rises.*

This is normally true, but sometimes when you add a small amount of carbs, particularly from a sweet-tasting source, it seems that your pancreas overreacts and kicks out more insulin than it needs to. The end result is that your blood sugar may actually drop somewhat from where it was before the meal. I have noticed this enough times that I know it to be true, at least in my case.

This ten-point drop was good news for me in a couple of ways. First, it clearly indicates that my pancreas works; it still functions pretty well and is quite capable of releasing insulin to respond to the intake of carbohydrates. Second, the results of the muffin plus Halo meal revealed that I can make this a normal part of my breakfast repertoire. I can enjoy the muffin and the little mandarin orange without feeling guilty or wondering if my blood sugar is running amok.

SAUSAGE, EGG, AND CHEESE MUFFIN WITH AND WITHOUT CLEMENTINE TEST		
	Muffin Alone	**Muffin with Clementine**
Before Eating	102	109
After 1 Hour	107	99
Total Blood sugar Rise	5 mg/dl	-10 mg/dl

Summary: This test demonstrated that, at least for me, it is possible to add a sweet, vitamin C–loaded clementine to a meal I knew was safe and still keep my blood sugar in good shape. Yeah!

Omelet Test: Part 1

Another breakfast I wanted to test was that famous American standard: the omelet. Who doesn't love omelets?

Omelet Test

Omelets are made from eggs, and if all you eat is an omelet, or perhaps add a little cheese and sausage, almost no type 2 diabetic has anything to worry about. If you were hungry enough, and had no worries about the calories, you could eat two or three or four and still not have to worry about your blood sugar rising. One problem with omelets, however, is that they don't seem quite right on their own. We normally like to enjoy a piece of toast with them, or maybe a biscuit covered with milk gravy.

As with the muffin test, I scheduled two separate days to test two similar but not identical meals. For the first meal I had a standard omelet, with cheese and bits of sausage inside. To make it more appealing, I added a low-carb muffin (around 5 grams of carbs) topped with sugar-free jelly (3 more grams of carbs). My blood sugar before the breakfast registered 104. One hour after the very filling meal, the monitor revealed my blood sugar had risen to 108, a scrawny little four-point rise. I had eaten a tasty and filling breakfast, and even with my insulin resistance, had only experienced a peak of 108 mg/dl. I was definitely within the safe range. Once again, this was no surprise. I fully expected good results, and I got them. There just weren't enough carbs involved in this meal to set my blood sugar racing skyward.

BASIC EGG OMELET WITH CHEESE AND SAUSAGE TEST	
	Dennis
Before Eating	104
After 1 Hour	108
Total Blood sugar Rise	4 mg/dl

Summary: No surprises here. There was little blood sugar rise. How could there be with so few carbs in this meal?

Omelet Test: Part 2

Next, I tried a "nutritionally enhanced" omelet.

Egg and Veggie Omelet

That first omelet meal had been enjoyable and filling, but there was one problem with it: it hadn't been particularly nutritious. It contained plenty of protein but few vitamins and nutrients. The question was this: "Was there a way for me to enhance the nutritional value of this meal significantly without a corresponding rise in blood sugar?" Of course I could have added a mango and a peach and accomplished this, but this would have added over 60 grams of carbs to the meal and created a blood sugar disaster.

So I turned to the vegetables. For my next meal my wife, Benedicta, joined me in the test. We both had an omelet as before, plus a low-carb muffin. But this time we jammed that omelet with bits of green pepper, tomatoes, onions, and lots of spinach. The combination of flavors made the omelet more interesting and enjoyable. It was a pleasure to eat. The only question was, how would this affect my blood sugar? Keep in mind that vegetables are not no-carb foods the way eggs and meat are. All vegetables have carbs, but most of them have relatively few carbs (potatoes and corn being two notable exceptions). So I was clearly upping the carb content of my omelet, but could my body tolerate this somewhat higher-carb omelet? Was this safe for me? Could I add this to my list of acceptable breakfasts?

Thankfully the results showed that I could. Benedicta started out at 96 before the meal (fasting blood sugar) and one hour afterward it rose to 102, a six-point rise. Perfect! Of course, her metabolic efficiency is much better than mine.

In my case, my blood sugar was at 109 before the meal, and one hour after finishing my last bite of that omelet and low-carb muffin it had once again dropped—this time to 98, an 11-point decrease! Wow! I had another great breakfast to add to the list. As compared with the previous sausage and cheese omelet, we had raised the nutritional level tremendously. There was a significantly higher level of nutrients in the second omelet, with no worries as to crazy fluctuations in blood sugar.

SAME EGG OMELET AS BEFORE BUT WITH ADDED VEGETABLES TEST		
	Dennis	Benedicta
Before Eating	109	96
After 1 Hour	98	102
Total Blood sugar Rise	-11 mg/dl	6 mg/dl
Summary: We added a significant amount of vegetables, had a more nutritious breakfast, and still our numbers were great! Now that's exciting!		

Why had Benedicta's blood sugar risen slightly while mine dropped 11 points after this second meal? Everyone's pancreatic functions and response to carbs and sugars are slightly different. My pancreas has always tended to be an "overreactor." When it senses carbs and sugars hitting the stomach, it seems to go into panic mode: "Oh no! Carbs and sugars! Quick, send out the emergency team. Dump out insulin, and more insulin, and let's get this situation under control—pronto!" The result is that in some cases when I add a few extra carbs to a low-carb meal, my blood sugar levels drop rather than rise.

You might say, "Well, if that is the case, why not add more carbs still? Why not add a large apple, a mango, and a couple of bananas?" Because I have found by experience and testing that there is a limit to the number of carbs my body can safely process. Adding a few extra carbs to a low-carb meal is no problem, but adding a lot of carbs to a low-carb meal turns it into a high-carb meal—and that definitely *is* a problem for me, and anyone else who is prediabetic or diabetic. Additionally, the more carbs you ingest, the more insulin is secreted. And high levels of insulin are exactly what we do not want. We must understand that high blood sugars are toxic to us, and so also are high insulin levels!

Remember that our objective in eating is not merely to record low numbers after every meal. After all, if I simply wanted low numbers, I could eat steak and eggs for breakfast, fish and eggs for lunch, and chicken and eggs for supper all my life and never have to worry about testing my blood sugar or having high blood sugar numbers ever again. But I would not be getting all the nutrition that my body requires. Our Creator has made all kinds of beautiful vegetables to grow out of the ground that are incredibly beneficial for us. And we must take advantage of them and eat them often for optimum health. There is a tendency, when you first realize what carbs and sugars do to your blood sugar, to simply want to play it safe and overindulge on meat and eggs. But there is no need for that, nor would it be beneficial. We must look to the vegetables and make them an important part of our diets.

The Power of Salads

When you think about nutrition for the diabetic, you cannot help but consider the salad. In some people's eyes, a salad is a lowly food item, something to be eaten quickly before you get to the real food. But for the diabetic, salads are vital. They are filled with nutrition, and they do little to raise your blood sugar, assuming you fill them with the right ingredients. For the diabetic, salads are the "new potatoes." In the old days you used French fries, mashed potatoes, fried potatoes, and baked potatoes to supplement your steak, fish, or whatever you considered your main dish. But the enlightened diabetic now makes salads his go-to filler.

Salads come in many varieties, but one of the best salads for diabetics is the chef's salad. These salads typically contain an egg, lettuce, ham or turkey, tomatoes, and several more vegetables. Unless you add croutons, there is not really a high-carb food to be found, which makes them ideal. In my case, I can eat a huge chef's salad and barely raise my blood sugar, usually no more than 15 or 20 points. (Regarding salad dressing, consider olive oil, Italian, or a low-sugar ranch dressing. But with ranch, be careful. Some ranch dressings are much higher in carbs than others.) I can fill myself up until I can't eat any more and still know that my blood sugar is behaving itself. You can't beat that.

The Wonderful Chef's Salad

I wanted to record an official test of the chef's salad for posterity's sake (and for yours), so I sat down for lunch one day with my blood sugar monitor in hand. Before the meal my blood sugar tested at 105. After enjoying my salad and waiting an hour after finishing, my second test revealed a 103. In this case my blood sugar never rose at all, at least not when I checked it when it should be peaking after the meal. The decrease of two points means essentially that there was no rise. In other words, nothing much happened.

That's exciting news, and it confirms that salads are the diabetic's friend. They just don't do much to raise blood sugar. This little test proves something I've known for years. And once I discovered this it totally changed my life and gave me all kinds of hope. Here's the point: It is definitely possible to eat a large meal, become filled and satisfied, get plenty of nutrition, and yet keep your blood sugar from rising much at all. All you diabetics who struggle constantly with high numbers ought to be shouting, cheering, and clicking your heels together (if you can manage it) at this point. And what that means is, there is hope for you! You are not doomed, it turns out. Diabetes is not so tough, not so powerful, not so deadly that it cannot be thoroughly whipped! But changes will have to be made.

LARGE CHEF'S SALAD WITH ONE EGG, LETTUCE, TURKEY, AND VEGGIES TEST	
	Dennis
Before Eating	105
After 1 Hour	103
Total Blood sugar Rise	-2 mg/dl
Summary: What a blessing! I enjoyed a nice meal, left the table filled and satisfied, and still my blood sugar was unmoved. Life is good!	

High-Carb Salads

Not all salads are low carb. It all depends upon what you put in them. Some people like to fill them with fruit, and that will raise the carb content significantly. Some scatter blood sugar–raising croutons all over them, spoiling them and making them problematic. Or sometimes people will eat a salad and then ruin the meal with a couple of slices of thick French bread. After my outstanding results with the chef's salad, I wanted to test myself after eating a relatively high-carb salad and see the difference. So I went to Walmart and checked out all their salads, turning them upside down to read their nutritional labels pasted on the bottom. The salad with the dubious honor of containing the highest amount of carbohydrate was the Thai Mango Salad, which came in with 50 grams of carbs, which is higher than what you would find in a normal-sized candy bar or a 12-ounce regular soda.

The salad was enjoyable and derived its carbs primarily from the mango pieces, an ample helping of dried, crispy chow mein–type noodles, and a fairly sweet salad dressing that came with it. It definitely had a sweeter taste than the chef's salad. One rule of thumb is, the sweeter the taste, the higher the sugars and carbohydrate levels.

Of course, this isn't true with diet, sugar-free products, but otherwise, if what you're putting into your mouth tastes sweet, there is a good reason for that: Sugar is involved.

My wife, Benedicta, joined me in this meal and test just for fun. Before the meal, her blood sugar was fairly high for a normal person, 107 mg/dl. After eating this 50-grams-of-carbs salad and waiting an hour, her blood sugar was 104. Though she had been a bit high at the beginning, her pancreas and blood sugar processing system worked beautifully and had everything under control in an hour's time. Good job, pancreas!

When I tested myself before the meal, I started out lower than Benedicta (go figure!). My blood sugar was at a comfortable 93, but an hour after that salad, it had risen to 129. This represented a 36-point rise, but it still left me below the 140 mark, which I consider my absolute limit. I had expected a higher number, but I have learned that there will always be surprises when you frequently do tests like these. In this case it was a pleasant surprise. Had it not been for this test, I never would have eaten this salad, and probably won't be eating it in the future, but I was gratified that I could handle these 50 grams of carbs in this meal and still remain on the safe side.

THAI MANGO SALAD (50 GRAMS OF CARBS) TEST		
	Dennis	Benedicta
Before Eating	93	107
After 1 Hour	129	104
Total Blood sugar Rise	36 mg/dl	-3 mg/dl

Summary: At one hour my blood sugar had risen 36 points; my wife's had decreased by 3. Still, neither of us hit 130, and that's not too bad. I can handle salad carbs a whole lot better than candy carbs, soda carbs, or bread carbs. Fifty grams of candy bar carbs or soda carbs would have sent my blood sugar into orbit, but 50 grams of salad carbs (at least this salad) produced far less of a spike.

After ingesting 50 grams of carbs in the salad, why was my peak relatively low? I have had 12-ounce sodas with around 40 grams of carbs and seen my blood sugar shoot up to the 170s. But here, ingesting more carbs, my blood sugar rose to a relatively benign 129. The answer has to do with fiber, which we discussed earlier in chapter 3. When you drink a soda or eat a candy bar, you are getting lots of sugar and very little fiber. A regular-sized Snickers bar contains about 1 gram of fiber per candy bar while carrying 33 grams of carbs. Sodas have virtually no fiber at all, and usually around 40 grams of carbs (for 12 ounces—and who drinks a mere 12 ounces anymore?).

But in the case of the 50-gram salad, there is a significant amount of fiber, and when you are taking in fiber along with carbs, the process your body uses to break down those carbs is slowed down. The result is a kinder, gentler experience, which gives your pancreas more time to do its job and with less stress. As a result, you will not see those terrible blood sugar spikes that you would see from candy, soda, doughnuts, and so forth.

What this means is that you can "get away with" more carbs from a high-fiber food or group of foods than you could with a low-fiber food, even though both may have an equal amount of carbs. And sometimes the high-fiber food will leave you with better numbers, even when possessing more carbs than the low-fiber food. Thus, a 50-grams-of-carbs salad leaves me with significantly better numbers than a 40-grams-of-carbs soda.

Richard Clark

A while back I was in the Houston area doing some ministry at a church there. I am always looking for an opportunity to talk with diabetics, and if possible interview them and conduct a blood sugar test or two with them. I asked the pastor if he knew any diabetics who might be willing to talk with me. He thought he did and sent over a man who introduced himself as Richard Clark. Richard is an electrician and also serves as the worship leader for the church. He had a fascinating story to tell.

Richard's mother had suffered terribly from diabetes some years before, and he had learned a lot about the disease from his mother's experience. Eventually she had both her legs amputated, she experienced kidney failure, and she had several heart attacks and a quadruple bypass. She finally died from the complications of diabetes. Richard had a brother who died from diabetic complications as well. This man definitely had a family history of diabetes.

Then it became his turn. Richard had been feeling terrible but wasn't sure what was wrong. He felt weak and fatigued and found himself constantly thirsty. He wondered if he wasn't suffering from diabetes, but being a hardy, independent kind of guy, he put off going to the doctor as long as he could. Finally, he was feeling so bad he had no choice but to make an appointment. The doctor ran some tests and told Richard that his blood sugar level was over 400 mg/dl! This is incredibly high. Slightly elevated blood sugar can bring about problems, but often it will take years for those problems to surface. But blood sugar over 400 can destroy you in a very short time. The doctor informed Richard that he was clearly diabetic. The monster that had ruined and shortened his mother's life and killed his brother was now at his doorstep.

Richard was scared. And with fear came motivation. He went back to his house and threw out all the ice cream and soda. He went cold-turkey away from sweets and embraced a diet of garden salads and grilled chicken breasts. His drink of choice became water. He was so determined to change his lifestyle and avoid the fate of his mother that he lost nearly 50 pounds over the next two months. He bought a glucose monitor and began checking his levels a couple of times each day. His goal was to get his blood sugar around 100, and over time he began to see those numbers show up on his monitor.

When Richard returned to the doctor, his results shocked his physician. He declared that he rarely saw diabetic patients who experienced such a dramatic improvement over such a short time. Richard's story is a powerful message of hope for all of us! He went from a blood sugar of more than 400 to getting his blood sugar in the low 100s simply by changing the foods he allowed into his mouth, and his diabetes essentially "went away." Of course, it could come right back if he went back to his previous diet, but he is not about to do that. Having seen his mother suffer so terribly from diabetes gave Richard a motivation and determination that many diabetics seem to lack.

Richard's Test

I love to do blood sugar tests! (I know I'm a little weird that way, but they have been such a help and inspiration to me!) While I was talking with Richard, I asked him if we could do a couple of post-meal blood sugar tests after two very different meals. He agreed, so that evening he came over and ate meal number one: a meal consisting totally of fruit. Before eating his meal, his blood sugar read 94—a great number, especially for someone who had been in the 400s a few years ago. For his meal, I gave him two big bananas, one large apple, and a mango. He enjoyed the fruit, and afterward we sat around and talked for an hour while we waited to see what the fruit was going to do to his blood sugar. One hour after he had finished the meal he tested himself again, and this time the monitor read 199. This represented a 105-point rise in about an hour's time!

Richard was surprised. He knew about cutting down on sugar and even starches but had somehow assumed that fruit would pose no problem for him. But fruit can surely be a problem! Anyone with blood sugar hovering around 200 is not in a good position.

I invited him back over the following evening for a second and a contrasting meal. Whereas the first night was "fruit night," the second evening was "veggies night." I provided him a chef's salad I'd purchased from Walmart, but to beef it up a bit, I had him cut up about half a green pepper and mix it in with the salad. As with the previous night, his before-meal blood sugar was outstanding—96 mg/dl. Once again, he ate the meal, waited one hour, and then tested himself. But this time the results were radically different. One hour after eating the salad, his blood sugar stood at 116—a scrawny little

20-point rise. Richard's comment on the two tests was simple and to the point: "The fruits were actually driving my sugar levels higher than I could ever imagine…I've learned a lesson through all of this—a really good one!"

RICHARD CLARK: FRUIT MEAL VS. VEGETABLE SALAD TEST		
	All-Fruit Meal	Chef's Salad
Before Eating	94	96
After 1 Hour	199	116
Total Blood sugar Rise	105 mg/dl	20 mg/dl

Summary: The proof is in the numbers. The four-fruits meal raised Richard's blood sugar significantly, but the chef's salad, with extra green pepper, raised it just slightly.

Test Summary

It was a simple test and the outcome was exactly what I expected, based on what I've seen in my own body over the years. The plain truth is that as healthy as fruit is, and as many vitamins as it typically has, fruit will raise the blood sugar of diabetics in a way that most vegetables never will. So the question is this: If one meal raises your blood sugar to 200, and with another meal your blood sugar never goes above 120, which type of meal might be better to focus on for diabetics and prediabetics? In Richard's case, with fruits versus vegetables, it was 199 (fruits) versus 116 (vegetables). Talk about the ultimate no-brainer!

You may say, "Yeah, but I'm not about to eat four pieces of fruit at one meal." No, probably not, but in many meals you may be ingesting all kinds of other sources of carbs, such as potatoes, bread, rice, pasta, and so forth. And by adding fruit to the mix, you are bumping up your carbs and your blood sugar levels even more. Now, the goal is not to say, "I'm never going to eat fruit again." In limited sizes and quantities fruit can be a nutritious part of your diet. But we need to see that fruit can be a significant factor in runaway blood sugar. When you look at a cake, or a pie, or mashed potatoes, or a soda, you ought to be saying to yourself, "Too much of this can really raise my blood sugar." And when you look at fruit, you ought to be saying *the exact same thing*!

One thing you will have to face if you are going to conquer your blood sugar woes is that people like you (and me) simply cannot eat the way other people eat. What others can get away with, we most definitely cannot. We cannot load massive amounts of carbs into our stomachs and assume all will be well. Let us, therefore, determine to manage our diets well, and to limit our carbohydrates wherever we can. I know I seem to pick on fruit a lot, but the refined, processed carbs are far worse: sugar (the number one bad guy, supreme over all dietary villains), white flour, white rice, white potatoes, corn chips, potato chips, and nearly all desserts and sweet pastries. By slashing these from our diet, we will be the better for it, and we may well live longer and be healthier than others who have never worried about or even thought about blood sugar.

The Big Four Starches

In the 1500s and the 1600s, quite a few European researchers were known as alchemists. They researched and experimented constantly in an attempt to try to convert lead into gold. They assumed that lead and gold were made up of the same elements, just arranged in a different fashion and in different measures. They reasoned that if they could somehow rearrange lead by some process or another, the lead would be converted to pure gold. It was a great theory, but it was based on a false assumption. Lead and gold are entirely different elements, and regardless of what is added, subtracted, melted, or rearranged, lead was never going to become gold.

There is, however, a conversion that goes on in our bodies every day. I am talking about the conversion of carbohydrate-containing foods into sugar in our stomachs. Actually, your body is so eager to accomplish this conversion it doesn't even wait for the food to hit your stomach. You have enzymes in your saliva that go to work on starches while they are still in your mouth as you chew your food. This process is natural, and we were created to do this, so we should not gasp in horror and ask, "What is wrong with me? I'm making sugar."

Metabolic Inflation

Our bodies are created as a type of converter—foods turn into sugar, and sugar supplies energy. If we manufacture too much sugar, we have a gland called the pancreas that quickly dispatches insulin to regulate the amount of sugar in our blood and to "escort" our blood sugar into cells that need it. This ensures that our bloodstream has neither too much nor too little sugar. So far, so good.

The problem lies with the fact that as we age our bodies become less and less efficient at processing the sugar we make. The pancreas has to essentially huff and puff and pump itself crazy just to keep up with the ever-increasing demands our overweight, sluggish, inefficient, untoned bodies are making upon it. It takes more and more insulin to get the job done. It is like a metabolic inflation. What we used to be able to purchase for $2 now costs $200. When inflation soars too high, we get to the point where we can no longer keep up. This is the essence of type 2 diabetes.

Add to this the fact that we are taking in far more carbohydrates now than at any time in man's history. Our early ancestors had no bagels, doughnuts, cake, ice cream, candy bars, sliced white bread, breakfast cereal, sodas, and the like. Much of their food supply was gained by hunting, fishing, picking berries, and growing vegetables. They enjoyed fruit in season but did not have an endless perpetual supply of it the way we do today. Nor was the fruit of those days genetically modified, as it is today, to make it far sweeter. Our ancestors were, in essence, low-carbers when low-carb diets had never been heard of.

The result of our weakening bodies, a genetic predisposition, and a preponderance of high-carb foods in our diets, and especially the ingestion of megadoses of sugar is the diabetes epidemic we see today.

Foods are made up of three macronutrients: fats, proteins, and carbohydrates. That's it—there are no more. Fats do virtually nothing to raise blood sugar. Proteins can raise it slightly. But carbohydrates are a different story. Carbohydrate-rich foods drive blood sugar up like nothing else. If you are diabetic and you find that your blood sugar is soaring into the 200s, 300s, or higher, you can bet the farm that your sugar levels didn't get that way by eating steak and salads! High blood sugar nearly always (and I could probably leave out the word *nearly*) results from the ingestion of significant numbers of carbs and sugar (which is a carbohydrate—the very worst offender).

Outstanding Blood Sugar Raisers

Certified diabetes educator Franziska Spritzler states:

> The total carbohydrate content of a meal is the most important in raising blood sugar after meals…Low-carbohydrate diets consistently outperform low-fat diets and even low-glycemic-index diets.[1]

Jenny Ruhl, diabetes researcher and author of the book *Blood Sugar 101*, writes:

> It is the carbohydrates you eat that raise blood sugar after meals. Sugars and starches. Nothing else. The fats you eat do not raise blood sugar at all.[2]

I would add that high-protein foods can raise blood sugar a bit, but for most type 2 diabetics, that rise will be so minimal and so stretched out over many hours it will be negligible. Foods with few carbs, such as meat, spinach, cucumbers, celery, and eggs, do almost nothing to raise blood sugar in normal people and type 2 diabetics. This is precisely what your blood sugar monitor will tell you again and again and again if you use it for post-meal tests. This truth is so evident and irrefutable that the only ones who could ever deny it (and believe me, some do!) would be those with a dietary ax to grind. These folks are so biased against a low-carb approach that they refuse to accept the obvious.

In a practical sense, high-carb, blood sugar–spiking foods can be divided into two groups: sugary foods and starchy foods. Both raise blood sugar very rapidly. And it is this point that deceives millions of diabetics and leads to their downfall. The association between sugary foods and high blood sugar is so well known that hardly anybody needs to hear it. We all know that a huge piece of pie liberally covered with ice cream is going to raise your blood sugar significantly. Most will agree that we cannot eat three candy bars for breakfast and expect to keep our blood sugar low. But while this is common knowledge, many do not recognize or ever consider that a large bowl of oatmeal and a couple of slices of Texas Toast can do the exact same thing!

The Big Four Starchy Blood Sugar Raisers: Bread, Pasta, Potatoes, and Rice

There are four types of foods I call the Big Four starches, which can be a real problem for diabetics. The Big Four include bread, pasta, potatoes, and rice. While everybody knows that diabetics have no business eating sugary foods and drinks, many seem to be unaware that these big four starches, along with some other starchy foods, are equally problematic. Many diabetics faithfully abstain from pie, cake, ice cream, and candy bars but think nothing of eating huge mounds of rice, large chunks of bread, or generous portions of mashed potatoes. And then they wonder why they are having so much trouble keeping their blood sugar levels in line!

Now, it's not that there are no other starchy foods that will do this to you, but at least for Americans, these four are the most popular and beloved starches. Just eliminate these foods from anyone's diet, and they would be almost certain to lose weight and improve their A1C scores in a major way.

Health and food writer Laura Dolson writes,

> Starches are long complex chains of simple sugars. This is why they are often called "complex carbohydrates." It was once thought that complex carbohydrates do not raise blood sugar as quickly or as much as sugars, but now we know that some starches are actually more glycemic than some sugars. In this sense, they are not "complex" for very long at all. People who are sensitive to sugar should avoid most starchy foods as well since most starchy foods are rapidly broken down into sugar.[3]

Doing What It Takes

In this chapter we will take a look at each of these food categories, note their inherent dangers for diabetics, and consider possible alternatives. At first glance, many would think that the elimination of bread, pasta, rice, and potatoes would be "a bridge too far." They might even declare that life would hardly be worth living if they eliminated these great-tasting staples of the American diet. The good news is that the most popular of these four, bread, does not really require total elimination for most type 2 diabetics. But whether you can find satisfactory substitutes or alterations, one thing is sure: if diabetics do not deal with reducing these "big four starches," they are facing a dismal future where their quality of life will be significantly reduced, and their years will, in all likelihood, be shortened. Is having potatoes or bread at every meal really worth that?

At the heart of any plan to conquer diabetes and runaway blood sugar must be this simple thought: *I will do whatever I need to do to get my blood sugar levels back down into the normal range.* This will lead to different steps for different folks, depending upon the level of severity of your diabetic condition, a condition that built up through decades of stuffing yourself with carbs, carbs, and more carbs. Not only does this lifestyle lead to an overworked, exhausted, ineffective pancreas, it also has created a constant state of hyperinsulinemia—the condition of having high levels of insulin in your bloodstream. Even if your blood sugar tests reveal normal levels, high insulin levels that result in ten times as much insulin in your blood as normal create serious health issues, in addition to making it almost impossible for you to lose weight.

Bread

Bread is so...lovable! It's comforting, it's sweet to the palate, it's filling, and meals just don't seem quite right when at least some member of this big family is not present. Bread is such a huge part of meals that in the Bible bread was often used in place of the word *meal*: instead of saying, "they ate dinner," you read that they "took bread" (Matthew 26:26). And when Jesus told us to pray, "Give us this day our daily bread" (Matthew 6:11), He probably wasn't talking just about bread, but the food we need to live and be healthy.

Understanding that bread raises blood sugar almost as rapidly and efficiently as table sugar, the question might be asked, "Why not just give up on bread altogether?" It's a good question. We do not become horribly sick and keel over dead because we don't eat bread. We can actually do quite nicely on a no-bread diet. If you were to reply that we need the carbs bread supplies to turn into sugar and supply energy to our bodies, you would be wrong. It is arguable that we even need carbs at all, but we certainly don't need bread carbs. You can get all the carbs you need from a garden salad or an avocado or peanuts or beans. Nearly all foods apart from meat will have some carbs. There is absolutely no reason why we must eat bread. It's not especially nutritious compared with vegetables. Why not just chuck out all our bread and never taste it again?

The answer to this question is that most of us would feel cheated and deprived if we thought we had to go through our remaining years without ever tasting bread again. And people who feel deprived and cheated are the ones who are most likely to end up forsaking their diet and going back to where they were before. My philosophy is this: Why should I give up something I don't have to? There are unquestionably some sacrifices I have to make to achieve normal blood sugar, and those I will gladly make. But I don't have such a martyr complex that I am going to sacrifice any food or treat not standing between me and good health just for the sake of being a purist.

Lots of Substitutes

Out of the "big four" starches, bread has the most pleasing and numerous possible substitutions and acceptable forms. There are seemingly infinite alternatives to normal, high-carb bread that still look like bread, smell like bread, and even taste like bread. And this is because they are bread, but not the kind of bread your momma fed you as a child. Nearly everyone on our planet has been brought up to eat bread and to consider it natural, normal, and a routine part of nearly every meal. Toast, sandwiches, hamburger and hot dog buns, tortillas, pizza crust, biscuits, muffins, and dozens of other bread products have been a part of our lives since we can remember. To suddenly and drastically cut all forms of bread can be a radical and traumatic step.

Don't mistake me—if that is what it would take for me to keep my blood sugar at safe levels, I would gladly do it. But when you do a little research you discover that wiping bread from our diets is entirely unnecessary. We may have to pay a little more, or order from internet companies, or make it ourselves in our ovens, microwaves, and bread machines, but for most of us it is worth it. I believe that a major reason I have not backslidden from the low-carb lifestyle is the fact that I have discovered so many tasty alternatives to the foods I had to sacrifice so I don't feel the least bit cheated. I enjoy my meals and my diet. I do not struggle daily with an inner voice that whispers, "Go back to doughnuts and ice cream and French bread and lasagna." I never feel as if I'm on the verge of pigging out on a mountain of ice cream or a super-sized order of French fries. This is why I am spending quite a bit of time on the subject of bread. I want you to succeed, not just for a few months, but for a lifetime. And the more alternative foods you have at your disposal, the more likely it is that you will make it!

How Bread May Be Converted from High-Carb to Low-Carb

Two major actions in creating bread will turn normally high-carb bread into low-carb bread: 1) change the primary ingredient from wheat to some other grain or ingredient, and/or 2) increase the fiber. This can easily be done, either by bread companies or by individuals at home, following recipes created or discovered by others. What you don't find much of are really, really low-carb breads at your local grocery store (with about 2 net carbs). When low-carb was a little more fashionable in times past, you could find a few low-carb bread products, but most of these have bit the dust. In most cases, if you want some low-carb bread, you'll have to either order it or make it yourself.

Tortilla Time

The major exception are low-carb tortillas. I find these in nearly every grocery store. So here is a start for you. If you can't afford or don't want to take the time to order low-carb bread from internet companies, stock up on low-carb tortillas and enjoy them often. But I need more than tortillas. And not being independently wealthy or being willing to spend huge amounts of money for bread, this means I had to learn a few things about baking!

Low-Carb vs. Whole Wheat Tortillas

I am always curious about precisely how much better whole wheat bread products are than white. I know that whole wheat contains more nutrients than white (although bread is never going to be a major source of nutrients the way that vegetables are). But considering just how forcefully the experts tell us to go whole grain, I wanted to test one against the other just to see how much of a blood sugar decrease I am able get in switching from white to whole grain. I decided to pit low-carb whole wheat tortillas against white tortillas. And then for good measure I tested myself with low-carb tortillas. In each test I ate two tortillas and heated them in a microwave.

TORTILLA TESTS			
	Whole Wheat	Normal White	Low-Carb
Before Eating	101	101	90
30 Minutes After Eating	118	113	117
1 Hour After Eating	142	141	137
1.5 Hours After Eating	163	177	153
2 Hours After Eating	174	164	142
3 Hours After Eating	138	124	138
Total Blood sugar Rise	73	76	63

Summary: There wasn't much benefit in going from white to whole wheat in this test. The whole wheat tortillas were superior nutritionally, but in raising blood sugar it was a wash. The biggest surprise in this test was the fact that the low-carb tortillas didn't act too much like a low-carb food. Their label stated that they had only 4 net grams each. The total of 8 net grams of carbs should not have raised my blood sugar to a peak of 153! This made me dubious of the nutritional information on the package of this particular brand.

A Further Test

I admit I was puzzled by the significant blood sugar rise I had after the two low-carb tortillas (8 net carb grams total). I have tested myself with these tortillas, using two of them to make a low-carb pizza, and seen much lower numbers than what I saw here. I was so intrigued that in the evening I made myself another pizza, using two of the tortillas as a base, to see what kind of blood sugar rise I would get. I had much better numbers with the pizza that I did when I just ate the tortillas by themselves!

LOW-CARB TORTILLA PIZZA (2 TORTILLAS) TEST	
Before Eating	78
1 Hour After Eating	119
1.5 Hours After Eating	123
2 Hours After Eating	107
Total Blood sugar Rise	45

Summary: Now that was more like it! Even though the total blood sugar rise was higher than I would like, the peak was still at a respectable 123. By two hours I was down to a happy 107. Why did I do so much better this time? There seems only one reasonable explanation. Because of all the extra fat from the meat and cheese I put on the pizza, the carbs from the tortillas were not converted to sugar nearly so fast as they were when I ate the tortillas by themselves. This demonstrates the power of fat to reduce blood sugar spikes. Yay, fat!

In comparing the pizza test with the two-tortillas-alone test, it is clear that the worst possible scenario is to eat carbs alone. By adding fat and/or protein (but especially fat) to a fairly high-carb meal, you cut down significantly on your total blood sugar rise. Even though the pizza had more total carbs than the tortillas by themselves, the presence of fat greatly improved the effect upon blood sugar.

Quesadillas

Another use for low-carb tortillas is to make quesadillas. Quesadillas are fabulous, and in most cases the only thing that makes them problematic for blood sugar are the tortillas that go on the top and the bottom. Substitute low-carb tortillas, and quesadillas can be eaten and enjoyed without guilt! When you eat quesadillas, most of what's inside the two tortillas—chicken, steak, cheese—possess a miniscule amount of carbs and have very little blood sugar–raising capacity. Once you have replaced the normal tortillas with low-carb tortillas, you have converted your quesadilla from high carb to low carb.

Quesadilla Test

I wasn't much worried about my blood sugar levels when I ate a quesadilla made with low-carb tortillas. I knew the meat, cheese, green peppers, sour cream, and picante sauce would have a minimal effect on my blood sugar. The biggest consideration by far would be the tortillas that would hold the conglomeration together. And because the tortillas listed 6 net grams of carbs each, I knew those 12 total net grams of carbs were unlikely to send my blood sugar soaring.

I enjoyed the quesadillas immensely, waited the requisite one hour after eating, and tested myself. Sure enough, the quesadilla had had a limited effect upon my blood sugar, raising it from 82 to 102. A 20-point rise isn't insignificant, but any time your blood sugar peaks at 102 after a meal, you can be sure you are doing very well indeed. I wish that were my peak after every meal!

LOW-CARB QUESADILLA TEST	
	Quesadilla with 2 Low-Carb Tortillas
Before Eating	82
After 1 Hour	102
Total Blood sugar Rise	20 mg/dl

Summary: What a delight to be able to enjoy and indulge in a full-sized quesadilla and not have any worries about runaway blood sugar! I am so thankful that low-carb tortillas may be found in nearly every grocery store, and for reasonable prices. Every diabetic should be taking advantage of these treasures often. Whenever your blood sugar peaks just above 100, you know that all is well!

You can use these low-carb tortillas as a wrap to create a breakfast for yourself. Simply stuff it with scrambled eggs, various cheeses, some veggies such as green peppers, spinach, and onions, and you are in business. A little avocado wouldn't hurt a bit! Your blood sugar will probably have very little rise, and you are good until your next meal.

We're just scratching the surface here. It is amazing to think that with these relatively cheap little tortillas, which taste exactly like their big-brother, high-carb tortillas, you can enjoy all sorts of meals you either thought you had to skip, or you went ahead and ate and sent your blood sugar off to the races. No more! Go to your grocery store and buy yourself a package or two of these tortillas and start experimenting.

Making Your Own Bread

When it comes to low-carb alternatives for bread and many other food items, we truly live in the best of times. There may not be too many super-low-carb breads on the shelves of your local grocery store, but recipes and cooking demonstrations of low-carb breads, muffins, bagels, and other bread products of all kinds overflow on the internet and on YouTube. They are so plentiful that you will never be able to try them all even if you should live to be 199. But usually you don't have to go through too many recipes of a particular bread product to find one you are well satisfied with.

First, let's look at a simple bread loaf. Our ancestors baked bread in their ovens all the time. Today we find it more convenient to go to the store and buy a loaf of bread. But the bread companies have never seemed to figure out that if they made at least one low-carb bread and stocked it on grocery store shelves, there are enough of us low-carbers that we would make it an instant hit. So we have to go back to the way great-grandma made bread. But with some differences.

The main problem with normal bread is the flour that is used—common baking flour made from crushing wheat ever so finely. It makes for a great-tasting bread but is terrible for diabetics. Can other flours be used? Yes! You can find all kinds of flours to experiment with.

Paleo flour (a high-fiber flour which has about half the net carbs of regular flour) tastes almost exactly like regular flour, but it has far more fiber and ends up possessing about half the net carbs of regular flour. Soy flour has about a third of the carbs of normal flour. Coconut flour has fewer carbs, and almond flour has fewer still. Any bread recipe made with these flours is going to be kinder to your body than the blood sugar–spiking, colon-clogging white flour we have become used to.

The internet abounds with low-carb bread recipes using these and other flours. Try a few until you find one that satisfies you. Go to YouTube and type "low-carb bread," or "almond bread," or "keto bread," or "low-carb muffins or biscuits" in the search engine. One word of warning: Don't expect any of these breads to taste exactly like ordinary bread made of ordinary wheat flour. They each will have their own distinctive taste, and with my limited experience I have not yet found one quite as good as the homemade bread (high-carb) my mother used to make. Still, I am more than willing to endure a slight reduction in taste to keep my blood sugar in line.

One of the simplest, easiest, and quickest ways to have bread with your meal is to make it in your microwave—a process that normally takes about 90 seconds. Some years ago somebody came up with the idea of a "muffin in a mug." The idea was to put a little flour in a mug, along with some melted butter or cooking oil, an egg, a little baking powder, and a small amount of nonsugar sweetener. Stir everything together well, pop the mug in your microwave, bake it for 90 seconds, and voilà, a muffin in a mug. It seems as if those first recipes often were based mostly on flaxseed. You always got a nice rise due to the egg and baking powder, and you definitely had a bread product that was low carb. The trouble was, those flaxseed muffins didn't taste all that great, and you generally had to put on some sugar-free jelly to make them palatable.

Pick a Flour, Any Flour

But after a while people began to experiment with other types of flours and combinations of flour: almond flour, coconut flour, soy flour, Carbquik, Paleo flour, and so forth. And lo and behold, it turned out that this concept would work with about any type of flour-type substance you cared to put in your mug. With that egg cooking right there in the mug, you were bound to get a rise and a muffin-like creation.

The good news is that some of these other flours had a much better taste than those original flaxseed muffins. Someone came up with the idea of adding a bit of vanilla flavoring to the mix, which made them better still. Someone else thought of using about a tablespoon of sour cream, which made them moister. I haven't seen any recipe that calls for heavy whipping cream, but I tried this in place of cooking oil or melted butter, and I liked this version better still.

Some other creative folks got the bright idea of turning this muffin into a little cake. By adding a tablespoon of cocoa powder and throwing in some bits of sugar-free chocolate and some sliced almonds, and then adding a bit more sweetener, you can create a wonderful little chocolate "cake in a mug." Top it with some whipped cream (which is relatively low carb) and you have a great little dessert that does not have to apologize to its big high-carb brothers for its taste. Turns out, when it comes to bread-like creations in mugs, the sky's the limit.

As I thought about this, I realized this same concept could be used to make "bread in a bowl." Mix a couple of low-carb flours (such as soy flour and almond flour) in a square or rectangular microwave-safe container. Add salt, an egg, baking powder, and a little melted butter or cooking oil, stir well, and pop in the microwave. Because the mixture is spread out over a larger surface, it will not rise as high, but of course that is what you want with bread. I sometimes put some high-fiber beans over it (such as small red beans) and have an old-fashioned meal of bread and beans, a meal my blood sugar monitor tells me is safe.

You can use many different bread substitutions to complete your otherwise bread-less meals. One problem for some who first start the low-carb lifestyle is getting filled up. They have a piece of chicken and a generous helping of green beans on their plate. So far, so good, but they know this isn't going to satisfy their hunger. Of course, they could have large salads with every meal, but that gets old. But in just a couple of minutes you can add a low-carb bread muffin or some bread-in-a-bowl you baked in your microwave, and now it feels like the meal is complete.

Below are three sample recipes to get you started. But remember that you can experiment with all sorts of low-carb flours to your heart's content until you find muffins and breads that suit you. Some of the flours you might want to try are almond flour, coconut flour, soy flour, Carbquik baking mix, Paleo flour, and ground flaxseed.

Low-Carb Muffin-in-a-Mug

Ingredients: 1.5 T. soy flour, 1.5 T. almond flour, 1.5 T. heavy whipping cream, 1 T. nonsugar sweetener of your choice, ½ tsp. baking powder, ¼ tsp. salt, ¼ tsp. vanilla extract (if desired), 1 egg.

Directions: Spray a large mug with cooking spray. Place all the ingredients in the mug and stir vigorously until well-blended. Place in microwave for about 90 seconds. Done!

Low-Carb Cake-in-a-Mug
(Use same ingredients and directions
as above with these changes)

- Cut soy and almond flour to 1 T. and add 1 T. cocoa powder.
- Add 1 heaping tsp. sugar-free chocolate chopped finely.
- Add a handful of sliced almonds.
- Add 1 T. sour cream to make it moister and cake-like.
- You might want to add a little more sweetener to make it taste more like a dessert.
- Top with whipped cream, if desired.

Low-Carb Bread-in-a-Bowl

Ingredients: 1.5 T. coconut flour, 1.5 T. almond flour, 1 T. cooking oil, 1 packet nonsugar sweetener, ½ tsp. baking powder, ¼ tsp. salt, 1 egg

Directions: Spray a medium-sized microwave-safe container with cooking oil. Mix all ingredient in the bottom of the container thoroughly. Place in microwave for 90 seconds.

White vs. Whole Wheat

Perhaps one of the greatest disservices many doctors and nutritionists have done for the diabetic community is to leave the impression that if we simply change from white bread to whole wheat bread, all our problems are over. They constantly preach that white bread is horrible for you and should be illegal, but whole wheat bread is noble, righteous, healthy, trustworthy, loyal, helpful, friendly, courteous, kind, and all the rest of the Boy Scout's motto. There is some truth in this, but it is not the whole truth.

Whole wheat bread offers three advantages over white bread. It has more fiber, it is somewhat more nutritious, and it can spike your blood sugar less sharply than its white cousin. On the debit side, however, there are a couple of things we need to recognize. First, all bread is going to raise blood sugar for insulin-resistant diabetics. It is not that white bread raises your blood sugar and whole wheat does not. It is more that white bread raises your blood sugar a lot and whole wheat bread raises it somewhat less—sometimes. One factor in this equation is just how finely the bread company has pulverized the whole grains to make their whole wheat bread. The finer the wheat kernels are crushed, the more they will act like white bread. Extremely rough, coarse whole wheat bread is your best bet. If your whole wheat bread has almost as fine a texture as white bread, you are probably not gaining much. Nutrition researcher Kris Gunnars writes, "Most breads are made of pulverized wheat. They are easily digested and rapidly spike blood sugar and insulin levels, which can lead to the notorious blood sugar 'roller coaster' and stimulate overeating."[4]

In diabetic literature and diabetic recipe books you will often find the phrase "healthy, whole wheat bread." This phrase is highly misleading. The reason is simple. What makes diabetics different from nondiabetics is their inability to process carbs efficiently. They have become, to some degree, "carbohydrate intolerant." Their insulin resistance has reached such a level that the blood sugar produced by carbohydrates is never fully absorbed into the cells, and all that excess sugar in the blood runs through the bloodstream, wreaking havoc on cells and organs, creating all sorts of miseries that we label "diabetic complications."

Because these facts are incontrovertible, to eat large amounts of a food like bread (in its normal form), which is close to pure carbohydrate, is the height of folly. And to imply that by switching from white bread to whole wheat bread we have fixed all of this is nothing but insanity. Picture a crazy man who spends hours every day cutting himself with a large knife, creating wounds, scabs, and infections all over his body. You decide you can fix him by taking away his knife and giving him a slightly smaller knife. He still cuts himself just as before, but the wounds and scabs are smaller. You haven't exactly done him much of a favor.

60 Gram Sliced Bread Comparison Test

I decided to test my own blood sugar response to equal portions of whole wheat bread versus white bread. To really make the difference obvious, I knew I would have to consume a lot of bread, far more than I would ever eat in any possible situation. I looked forward to getting the results and taking all of this out of the realm of theory and into the cold, hard realm of numbers on my monitor. On the other hand, I dreaded the test, knowing that it would push my blood sugar way too high in both cases. Still, I felt I had to do it.

I started with the whole grain bread. The bread had 15 net grams of carbs per slice, so four slices equaled 60 grams of carbs. I toasted the bread and buttered it for taste, and then ate the bread, one slice after another. It was a lot of bread! Some people would say I had a healthy meal. After all, this bread had no animal fat; in fact, it had no fat at all. It had zero cholesterol and would be praised by many as a "heart healthy" meal. But there is nothing healthy for your heart when your blood sugar levels are soaring.

One hour after stuffing myself with all that bread, those 60 grams of (whole wheat) carbs drove my blood sugar from 103 before the meal to 176 at the one-hour mark. This is a dangerous level, and when rises like this become a normal part of your life, you are headed for disaster. This was well beyond my own self-imposed limit of 140. On to test #2.

In order to make the breads relatively equivalent, I ate four and a half slices of white bread because the white bread had only 13 net grams of carbs per slice. This should have made for around 60 grams of white bread. As before, the bread was toasted and buttered. One hour after eating my monitor read 202, which represented a 104-point rise (my pre-meal test was 98). The white bread did raise my blood sugar higher than the whole wheat, but both raised it to unacceptable and dangerous levels.

WHOLE WHEAT VS. WHITE BREAD TEST (60 GRAMS EACH)		
	Whole Wheat Bread	White Bread
Before Eating	103	98
After 1 Hour	176	202
Total Blood sugar Rise	73 mg/dl	104 mg/dl

Summary: Whole wheat bread, with its higher fiber, does tend to raise blood sugar less than white, at least in this test with these particular breads and my body. However, clearly both white and wheat raised my blood sugar far too high. Turns out that "healthy whole-grain" bread may not be quite as safe and harmless as some of the experts have been declaring.

Pasta

We Americans love our pasta. In my childhood years my family had countless dinners that revolved around macaroni and cheese and spaghetti. Never once did any of us give any thought to pasta's effects upon blood sugar. It was only after I faced the very real prospect of diabetes that I became aware that pasta was not my friend.

There is one thing that pasta has going for it, which is absent in bread, potatoes, and rice. Due to the way pasta is made, its sugars are locked more tightly together, and therefore pasta will tend to break down in your stomach a bit slower than most other starchy foods. This is a good thing and means that you may not get as much of a blood sugar spike with pasta as you would with a carb-equivalent amount of bread or potato. That being said, pasta is still a high-carb starch and should be either avoided or eaten in small quantities.

When you understand that pasta is not a friend of diabetics, you will start to avoid Italian restaurants, where the majority of their meals have pasta as a base. Sometimes this is just not possible, particularly when you are with a group of pasta lovers. In such cases where you are pressured to go to an Italian restaurant, do yourself a favor. Order a chef's salad and lose the croutons.

Spaghetti Tests

What could be more American than spaghetti? Yes, I know it didn't originate here, but we have surely adopted it as one of our go-to meals for dinner and sometimes for lunch. The only problem is those starchy noodles that make up the foundation for that marvelous sauce. There are all kinds of pasta, but their differences are mostly in shape. For our purposes we will use spaghetti and some potential substitutes to demonstrate possibilities for diabetics.

Plain Noodles Spaghetti Test

For this first test my wife, Benedicta, and I ate traditional, white spaghetti noodles. They tasted great, but I knew they would do a number on my blood sugar. Ben, who is far less insulin resistant than I am, didn't rise to my heights, even when she started out with a slightly higher blood sugar level. (Maddening, isn't it, how normal people can get away with so much more than we insulin-resistant types can?)

For our test, we measured one and a half cups of the cooked noodles, covered them with plain old spaghetti sauce (Ragu, not especially sweet), and then enjoyed the spaghetti. The numbers tell the story. My blood sugar rose a whopping 75 points, while Ben's rose only 20 points. Keep in mind that this was only spaghetti. Nobody eats only spaghetti. Often we have a large piece of bread with it, along with some other side dishes that would raise the carb levels still higher. And then, to add insult to injury, we have a sugary dessert to finish the meal. What this amounts to is a slow suicide by sugars and starches.

REGULAR SPAGHETTI NOODLES WITH SAUCE TEST		
	Dennis	Benedicta
Before Eating	84	111
After 1 Hour	159	131
Total Blood sugar Rise	75 mg/dl	20 mg/dl

Summary: Even though Ben started out quite a bit higher than I did, she ended up 28 points lower. But both of us, the normal and the not-so-normal, saw a blood sugar rise. Mine was significant; Ben's, not so much.

After this we went on to try several other types of pasta, noodles, and noodle substitutes.

Shirataki Noodles

Among the low-carb crowd, these noodles are frequently mentioned. They are not really noodles, at least not in the traditional sense. They are made from the konjac root and originated in Japan. They are packed in water, and the noodles you buy are about 97 percent water and the rest indigestible fiber. This means they possess essentially zero calories and zero net carbs. They don't do you much good, but they don't do you much harm either. But they do fill you up, and they do not raise blood sugar. The problem with this alternative to pasta is not really the taste. After you wash them in hot water for a few minutes, they have almost no taste at all. The problem is with the texture. They have a rubbery, gelatinous feel in your mouth, which I did not like at all.

SHIRATAKI NOODLES WITH SAUCE TEST		
	Dennis	Benedicta
Before Eating	99	102
After 1 Hour	111	109
Total Blood sugar Rise	12 mg/dl	7 mg/dl

Summary: Our blood sugar peaks were well within the acceptable level. In fact, we should have had lower numbers than this. I expect it was because Ben put a few vegetables in the sauce. Had we eaten these "noodles" without any sauce, our blood sugar probably would have stayed put, or even dropped a few points. But to eat them without sauce would have made me gag!

Dreamfields Noodles

The Dreamfields company has been making pasta for quite a few years now, and they used to make an interesting claim. For years they boasted that they had a unique process of treating their pasta that made most of it indigestible. They used to say a typical portion of their noodles would include 41 grams of carbs. However, they listed 31 of these grams as "protected carbs" and with 5 grams of fiber, that's only 5 grams of digestible carbs.

After a lawsuit, the Dreamfields company quit bragging about their protected carbs and simply state that their pasta is healthy, has more fiber than ordinary pasta (which is true), and can be part of a healthy diet.[5] When I first began encountering blood sugar issues, I tested myself with the Dreamfields pasta and found that they did tend to result in lower numbers than regular pasta, but not all that much lower.

Still, even if it can't live up to its initial boasts, if it can reduce blood sugar spikes by even 20 percent over regular spaghetti, that's not too bad. Ben and I tested ourselves with the Dreamfields spaghetti noodles, using the same type of sauce as before (Ragu Traditional) and here are our results.

DREAMFIELDS NOODLES WITH SAUCE TEST		
	Dennis	Benedicta
Before Eating	95	112
After 1 Hour	135	114
Total Blood sugar Rise	40 mg/dl	2 mg/dl

Summary: For some reason Ben's base blood sugar was running high during some of these tests, higher than my own. But she always ended up finishing lower than I did. My blood sugar rise of 40 was not insignificant, but my one-hour peak of 135 was much better than the 159 I had with regular spaghetti noodles. The Dreamfields pasta tastes exactly like regular pasta—there is no sacrifice in taste at all. But be careful: Some people report that Dreamfields pasta spikes their blood sugar just as much as regular pasta.

Spaghetti Squash

Here is my favorite low-carb spaghetti pasta substitute. Spaghetti squash requires baking, but the process is simple, and when you're done, you have what look like little angel hair noodles.

Directions: Start by cutting the squash in half. Smear some olive oil and sprinkle some salt on the two halves of the squash before baking at 400° with the halves facing down for 45 to 50 minutes. Once baked, score the surface of the squash with a fork, which will give you the "noodles."

Of course, this is not pasta, but it tastes quite good. This is a wonderful way to enjoy your favorite spaghetti sauce! It still has some carbs, so it is not a freebie, but it is far superior to regular pasta.

SPAGHETTI SQUASH TEST	
	Spaghetti Squash with Sauce
Before Eating	107
After 1 Hour	116
Total Blood sugar Rise	9 mg/dl

Summary: Any time your post-meal blood sugar peak is below 120, you know you are in good shape! I would imagine that the spaghetti sauce was probably responsible for at least half the blood sugar rise in this test. No, spaghetti squash doesn't have the same taste or texture as normal spaghetti pasta, but it's quite good, and after eating it regularly with your favorite spaghetti sauce, you will hardly miss the old-fashioned noodles. It does cost a bit more, but it's more than worth it for the gentle way it treats your body.

Spaghetti Using Zucchini Noodles

You can buy a spiralizer for about $15 in many stores or online, and turn zucchini into a spiral, noodle-looking heap. By putting your spaghetti sauce over a large heap of these zucchini noodles you can have low-carb spaghetti.

SPAGHETTI ZUCCHINI TEST	
	Zucchini "Noodles" with Sauce
Before Eating	105
After 1 Hour	119
Total Blood sugar Rise	14 mg/dl

Summary: Here is another viable alternative to using regular pasta with your spaghetti sauce. When you smother these zucchini spirals with sauce, you really don't taste the zucchini—you taste the sauce. Yet somehow the texture is so completely different from regular pasta that I didn't like them too much. I greatly prefer the spaghetti squash used as a base for my spaghetti sauce. As with the previous test, I would guess that the sauce was at least half responsible for the small blood sugar raise I saw. But to see my blood sugar peak at 119 was a beautiful thing!

White Versus Whole Wheat Pasta Test

Once again, I wanted to test to see if whole wheat really made a significant difference over white. Often when we buy whole wheat pasta, or whole wheat bread, or brown rice, we feel noble and wise, indulging in a little self-congratulation. All those other less-enlightened people buy the white bread or the white rice or the white pasta. We know better.

But does whole wheat pasta really have that much of an advantage over white when it comes to raising or not raising blood sugar? I know the few tests I've done don't forever settle the issue, but at least they will give us a little idea about this. For my first test I ate a cup and a half of cooked, regular white spaghetti noodles. For the second test I ate a cup and a half of whole wheat spaghetti noodles. The results were not exactly what most would predict.

WHITE SPAGHETTI NOODLES VS. WHOLE WHEAT NOODLES (1.5 CUPS) TEST		
	White Noodles	Whole Wheat Noodles
Before Eating	99	102
After 30 Minutes	137	124
After 1 Hour	141	159
After 1.5 Hours	136	164
Total Blood sugar Rise	42 mg/dl	62 mg/dl

Summary: The regular noodles didn't raise my blood sugar as high as I thought they would. But strangely, the whole wheat noodles raised my blood glucose higher than the white—20 points higher. Thirty minutes after eating, the whole wheat noodles didn't seem to be doing too much, but as time passed they kicked into high gear and went to work on blood sugar. This little test surely demonstrates that whole wheat products are not necessarily always superior to white in their capacity to raise blood sugar.

This test blows at least a small hole in the "healthy whole wheat" phrase that we hear so much about. Sure, in nutrition and fiber they are superior, but in their tendency to keep blood sugar down, not always! I am guessing that the reason the whole wheat noodles raised my blood sugar so much is that they are probably a heavier, denser noodle than the white, and so I was getting more mass even though I ate one and a half cups worth of both noodles. Had I measured the noodles by weight rather than by the one-cup measure, the results probably would have been more equal. But then, most people do not measure their food this way. The bottom line is that people who think they are doing their blood sugar levels a favor by going whole wheat may sometimes be mistaken.

Potatoes

While bread does have a bit of a reputation as a blood sugar raiser, many other starchy foods sneak by nearly everyone without being exposed for what they are and what they do. Take a baked potato for instance. Baked potatoes will break down into sugar in your mouth and your stomach and often raise blood sugar nearly as fast as if you had simply swallowed many teaspoons of pure table sugar. Nutritionist and food writer Laura Dolson writes, "Too often, glucose is associated with sweetness and regular white potatoes are not a food that's generally considered sweet. Potatoes are almost all starch, though, and that starch is made up of long strings of glucose. Since the starch in potatoes is rapidly digested, the glycemic index of potatoes can be almost as high as that of glucose alone."[6]

What this means is that what goes into the mouth tasting starchy and not the least bit sweet is converted into sweet, nasty, troublesome sugar inside your stomach with blazing speed. Within minutes of eating a potato you have a belly full of sugar, and that sugar will end up in your blood, driving your pancreas into a spasm, creating excessively high insulin levels and resulting in miserably high numbers on your blood sugar monitor when you test a little bit later.

Potato Test

To demonstrate this, I did something I had not done in probably over ten years: I ate a medium-large, regular white baked potato. I was so curious about exactly what it would do to my blood sugar that I did not wait an hour or even 30 minutes to test my blood sugar after the potato. I tested myself at 15 minutes, 30 minutes, 45 minutes, and then one hour after eating.

Later, I decided to do the same test with a similarly sized baked sweet potato. Sweet potatoes have a reputation for being lower on the glycemic index (they don't break down in your stomach as quickly), so I thought I would see what my blood sugar monitor had to say about sweet potatoes. I purchased a sweet potato that seemed to be about the same size as the russet potato and ran the test again.

REGULAR WHITE POTATO VS. SWEET POTATO TEST		
	White Potato	Sweet Potato
Before Eating	101	109
After 15 Minutes	108	112
After 30 Minutes	152	152
After 45 Minutes	184	160
After 1 Hour	195	184
Total Blood sugar Rise	94 mg/dl	75 mg/dl

Summary: The blood sugar rise I got from that white potato confirmed all I had read and heard about potatoes. This one potato, all by itself, gave me a major blood sugar rise. Who would think an innocent-looking baked potato could do such damage! The blood sugar rise from the sweet potato was a bit less, but it was still too much.

In some of the articles I read while researching white potatoes versus sweet potatoes I ran into all sorts of nonsense. One person, who worked for a plant-based, vegan magazine, declared that all whole foods, even the sweetest ones, are healthy and "safe" for diabetics. In her mind table sugar is bad and nasty, but if sugar comes in fruits or through starches—no problem. But the tests above prove that there is a *big* problem with starches, even if the foods are "whole." What she and so many other "experts" miss is that what makes a diabetic a diabetic is their inability to process carbs and sugars the way normal people do. A normal person would not get a 195 blood sugar level after eating a single potato. But I did! And since I don't react and respond to carbs and sugars the way normal people do, I cannot possibly eat the way normal people eat. If I was allergic to peanuts and they made me deathly sick, it would be stupid for me to continually stuff myself with peanuts, claiming the right to eat like everybody else. I am not everybody else—I am me! If peanuts make me gravely ill, I won't eat peanuts. And if baked potatoes launch my blood sugar into dangerous levels, I will not eat potatoes—period!

Another argument I heard from those defending potatoes went something like this: "Potatoes vary in their carbs and sugars and in how quickly they break down in your stomach. And the way you fix them will make a difference in glucose levels as well. Plus, what foods you eat with them can make a difference. So you really can't say much about them, one way or another." Excuse me for saying this, but this is a silly argument. By this reasoning, you could never say anything about any food. The answer is simple. In whatever form you prefer your potatoes—baked or boiled or fried, skins or no skins, with chicken or with steak—test yourself an hour after you finish your meal. If you get a 225, you know: "Houston, we have a problem." The next night eat that same meal minus the potato and see what your blood sugar reads an hour later. If after that meal you get a 125, you can be pretty sure the potato is the culprit. If you want to try a different type of potato or try fixing it a different way, go ahead. But be sure to test yourself to discover how your body is tolerating that meal. One thing is for sure. If you eat a steak, a garden salad, and a potato, any high blood sugar level you see on your monitor is not because of the steak or the garden salad.

Rice

Rice is another starch that is merciless in its passion to raise your blood sugar to incredibly high levels. And rice is sneaky. Its carbs add up even though those little rice kernels on your plate look rather harmless. They don't give away the terrible secret that they are incredibly potent in the carbs they contain and their ability to send your blood sugar soaring. For example, if you had three slices of large white bread on your plate, you would surely know you were dealing with a major attack on your blood sugar. But a cup of cooked rice contains about as many carbs as nearly three slices of bread and raises blood sugar almost as fast (for diabetics). And many people would never be satisfied with one cup of rice under their beef stew or stir-fried meal; they would want close to two cups of rice, equivalent to eating about five or five and a half slices of bread. To heap up a huge mountain of rice on your plate is an absolute blood sugar nightmare for anyone with insulin resistance, regardless of the savory food you may pile on top.

Like other starches, rice does not taste sweet when it is in your mouth (unless you have put sugar on it). And its nonsweet taste deceives many. But like the other starches, rice consists of sugar chains bound together, and those chains are just waiting for a little saliva and stomach acid to quickly unravel them and turn them back to pure sugar.

The type of rice you eat can make a difference in the speed at which the rice converts to sugar. Wild rice converts much slower than brown rice (although wild rice is not really rice, people eat it as rice). Brown rice converts slower than white rice. But the rice that converts to sugar with dizzying speed is instant white rice, which is rated 128 on the glycemic index. This rice is like Superman, who can change from a mild-mannered reporter to a superhero wearing tights and a cape in a second—provided there is a phone booth near. (By the way, where does he do this now that phone booths have disappeared?) Instant white rice is in such a hurry to change into sugar that it barely hits your stomach before emerging as full-scale sugar ready for action. But almost any rice is going to convert to sugar fairly rapidly, so don't suppose you can simply change from white rice to brown rice and all will be well.

Unlike bread, there are not nearly so many rice substitutes that will satisfy, but there are several of them to consider. Some people simply grind/chop various foods like cabbage into rice-sized pieces, put it under a stew, and call it rice. There is a "rice" made of shirataki. I haven't tried this, but if it is as nasty tasting as the noodles I ate several years ago, thanks, but no thanks.

The number one low-carb rice substitute is a simple creation made of cauliflower. You chop the cauliflower very fine in a food processor, put it in a covered pan, and cook it for seven or eight minutes in 1 to 2 tablespoons of cooking oil. Salt to taste. It isn't bad, and there are dozens of ways you can mix it with other low-carb foods to make a meal out of it. Still, it does not really taste like rice, so don't expect it to.

White Rice vs. Brown Rice

Is brown rice superior to white rice in terms of blood sugar? I had to test this for myself, and my wife, Benedicta, joined me in the two tests.

Rice Test – White vs Brown

First, we ate 1 cup of cooked white rice, and tested ourselves 30 minutes later and then at the one-hour mark. At 30 minutes Benedicta's blood sugar was at 112 and mine was at 157. By an hour both of our glucose levels had begun to fall a bit. (When you peak at 30 minutes and are going back the other direction by one hour, it indicates that this food converted to sugar very rapidly.) At one hour Ben's blood sugar had dropped to 99, while mine stood at 151.

That the rice raised my blood sugar significantly was no surprise to me. This is exactly what we might expect it to do to someone with blood sugar issues. But I wanted to see how the white rice would compare with brown rice. Would the brown rice prove any better? My level of 151 was not a huge number, but it was definitely too high and well past the normal range. Ben's level of 99 was just fine, but then, she is the normal one.

Later we repeated the same experiment with the brown rice, and the results were surprising. Benedicta's blood sugar rose more after eating the brown rice than it did with the white rice.

WHITE RICE TEST		
	Dennis	Benedicta
Before Eating	93	107
After 30 Minutes	157	112
After 1 Hour	151	99
Total Blood sugar Rise	64 mg/dl	5 mg/dl

Summary: A cup of white rice was enough to raise my blood sugar 64 mg/dl, which was a pretty significant rise. Considering that many people eat a larger helping than a one-cup serving with their meals and may have worse insulin resistance, rice is clearly a food to be wary of. Benedicta started out 14 points higher than I did but ended up 52 points lower. She clearly processes carbs much more efficiently than I do!

BROWN RICE TEST		
	Dennis	Benedicta
Before Eating	98	96
After 30 Minutes	117	137
After 1 Hour	141	107
Total Blood sugar Rise	43 mg/dl	41 mg/dl

Summary: My blood sugar response to the brown rice was about what most would expect—it raised my blood sugar significantly but not as much as the white rice had. Strangely, Benedicta, who processes carbs better than I do, ended up with worse blood sugar levels this time compared with the white rice. After one hour, her 107 was a decent number, but strangely, at the 30-minute point, my blood sugar rise was less than hers. I'm not sure what this proves, but one thing is for sure. Choosing brown rice is no guarantee that you will have no blood sugar rise. Any kind of rice is going to give your pancreas a serious workout, and if you are diabetic, you had better either watch your portion sizes carefully or do without.

Final Thoughts About Starches

Starches are the Achilles heel for many diabetics. Many people simply refuse to accept the idea that foods so thoroughly normal as bread, potatoes, rice, and pasta could be all that problematic. After all, everybody eats these foods constantly. *Momma served me these wonderful foods all through my growing-up years, and Momma surely couldn't be wrong! People have been eating starches since time immemorial.* To learn that they may be detrimental to your metabolic health is too much to believe. To complicate matters, numerous reports of vegan and plant-based "cures" of diabetes seem to work and allow people to eat as many starches as they want.

We will get to the vegan/vegetarian versus low-carb controversy later in the book, but for now let me simply say that your blood sugar monitor is not a liar, nor is it susceptible to bias or deception. It states what is going on in your blood at the time you test it. And anyone who will take the time to test their blood sugar about an hour after eating a lot of starches will find that they provoke high blood sugar in a way that garden salads, meat, green beans, nuts, and avocadoes never do. Anyone except nondiabetics. Of course, if you have excellent pancreatic function and zero insulin resistance, you may well be able to eat a mountain of rice, a large baked potato, and a fat chunk of bread and still have quite good blood sugar levels an hour later.

But you are not the ones who need to be reading this book. I am writing this book to share my experiences and give hope and encouragement to diabetics—people who have been told by their doctors that they had better get those blood sugar levels under control or they are in serious trouble, people who have tried different diets and made numerous attempts to find the answer and still have A1C scores of 7, 8, 9, or higher.

If you are in this category, you probably need to seriously consider finding alternatives for bread, pasta, potatoes, and rice, or at the very least strictly limit your portions when you do eat them. Test yourself after eating them to see what they are doing to your blood sugar. Almost certainly you will find that they are giving you significantly high numbers, just as they do me. After all, I am one of you! The only thing that stands between me and diabetes is my diet and the grace of God.

More About Bread

Although I discussed bread in the previous chapter, I want to go into a little more detail here and share some more tests and some bread substitutes with you. Bread is so important and such a vital aspect of nearly everybody's prediabetes diet that most of us really need to find a way to include bread in our meals while still achieving normal blood sugar.

When it comes to bread, we need to remember two essential truths: 1) Bread in most of the forms in which we Americans eat it is a metabolic time bomb and can raise blood sugar more rapidly than almost any other food except pure sugar (and even compared to sugar, it doesn't come far behind), and 2) there are ways to create breads (or purchase them already created this way) that will possess very little of this blood sugar–raising capability.

Why Bother?

But before we go on to further explore the subject of bread, I want to say a few words about why it is so important to keep your blood sugar levels down close to or in the normal range. I have to admit that in some ways, constantly testing my blood sugar before and after meals and foods seems like a game. And I have always had an extremely competitive streak. I like to win. So when I see high numbers show up on my blood sugar monitor, I know I have just lost that round. It feels terrible. On the other hand, when my blood sugar peaks out at no more than the low 100s, I feel great. I am a big winner!

But we need to see that checking our blood sugar and discovering the numbers that reflect how much sugar is in our blood is far more than a game. It has everything to do with our health, longevity, and future. Consistently high blood sugars spell doom, pain, misery, and all sorts of health complications for us in the future. Consistently normal blood sugars spell a bright future. Let's consider what some doctors and researchers have to say on this subject.

Registered dietician Joanne Rinker writes:

> Sugary blood has a thicker, stickier consistency. You can imagine how hard it can be for thick syrup to get to the tiniest point of small blood vessels—places like the eyes, the ears, the nerves, the kidney, the heart.[1]

When your blood fails to circulate as it should, you end up with all kinds of complications, including foot pain, eye damage that can lead to blindness, and the failure of various organs. The truth is, your blood was never meant to be filled with sugar and be syrupy. It is supposed to be watery and flow freely. But the higher your blood sugar levels rise, the more syrupy your blood becomes, and the more damage is being done, day by day, to your body and your organs.

The American Diabetes Association says this:

> Over time, high blood glucose levels can damage both blood vessels and nerves in your body. This can result in poor blood flow to your hands and feet in addition to your legs, arms, and vital organs. Poor blood flow to these areas increases your risk of infections, heart problems, stroke, blindness, foot or leg amputation, and kidney disease. In addition, you can either lose the feeling in your feet or have increased pain in your feet and legs. Damage to your feet can occur from mild injuries, and you may not know

it. Finally, damage to blood vessels and nerves can lead to sexual problems that are difficult to treat. For all these reasons, you should make a major effort to avoid high blood glucose levels in your body.[2]

Let me repeat that last sentence one more time: "You should make a major effort to avoid high blood glucose levels in your body."

On the National Kidney Foundation website, we read these words:

If your diabetes is not well controlled, the sugar level in your blood goes up...High blood sugar can cause damage to very small blood vessels in your body. Imagine what happens to sugar when it is left unwrapped overnight. It gets sticky. Now imagine how sugar "sticks" to your small blood vessels and makes it hard for blood to get to your organs. Damage to blood vessels occurs most often in the eyes, heart, nerves, feet, and kidneys.[3]

The deceptive thing about high blood sugar is that it doesn't happen immediately. It is not as though you eat a doughnut for lunch and by the evening your feet are killing you and you can barely see anything. You can get by with high blood sugar for some time, perhaps many years, and feel great. But chances are, sooner or later it is going to catch up with you. For some it only takes a couple of years of consistently high blood sugar; for others it may take a decade or longer. But it will get you.

A Big Deal

So when we do these blood sugar tests and demonstrate the foods that do or do not raise blood sugar, this is not just a cute little game. Blood sugar levels are tremendously significant and have extremely important consequences about your quality of life in future years, and indeed how many years you may have left. Every day that you keep your blood sugar levels near normal, you are buying yourself a brighter future and making the terrible complications of diabetes less likely to appear in your life.

Most of you reading this book have already lived a significant portion of your lives enjoying the luxury of eating whatever you liked. You filled yourselves with cake and ice cream, with pie and sugar-filled cheesecake, with rice and mashed potatoes and baked potatoes and large bowls of breakfast cereal and...well, you get the idea. You can't do anything about that. What's done is done. But you can do everything about the way you eat from the present moment until your final day on this earth. Putting together days, weeks, months, years, and decades of low-carb foods and meals and keeping your blood sugar levels close to normal is a small price to pay to enjoy good health and extend your years considerably. And getting a handle on this issue of bread is no small part of this.

In "The Basic Food Groups: Carbohydrate," Dr. Richard Bernstein provides us with important words to consider: "The ADA has recently recognized officially that...bread is as fast-acting a carbohydrate as table sugar...Whether you eat a piece of the nuttiest whole-grain bread, drink a Coke, or have mashed potatoes, the effect on blood glucose levels is essentially the same—blood sugar rises, fast."[4]

Now, this sounds depressing for those who love bread and are not too excited about giving it up altogether. But the good news is this: Not all bread is created equal. You can discover this easily with a quick trip to your local grocery store. The first thing you notice in the bread aisle is the huge number of choices of bread available. You find sliced bread in wheat, white, and whole wheat versions, not to mention English muffins, bagels, tortillas, and buns of various types. Bread is available in many different shades, some with little oat flakes on the sides and some with sesame seeds. You can find generic brands of sliced bread for less than a dollar and some breads costing over $3 or $4. But for the diabetic, the issue with bread is not how cheap it is or whether it has seeds or flakes sprinkled all over the outside. The issue comes down to carbohydrates and fiber.

Don't Be Naive

As you peruse the many breads on your grocery store shelf, the number one rule is this: don't be impressed by color, don't be impressed by flakes or seeds on the bread, and by all means don't be impressed by the various claims you see on the wrappers. One particular bread I found boasted that "two slices supplies 100% of your day's need for whole grain." But when you check out the carbohydrate count, you find that it has 20 grams of carbs per slice with 3 grams of fiber. That leaves 17 net grams of carbs per slice, which means that to eat a sandwich with this bread, using two slices, you will get as many carbs as you would by eating a candy bar. And the bread will turn into sugar almost as fast as the candy. But because the bread doesn't taste sweet, many people have no idea just what a load of sugar these healthy-looking pieces of bread are carrying.

One of the reasons diabetics can enjoy bread without a major rise in blood sugar is due to the fact that we have a whole lot more bread choices today than in any previous generation. Most of them you'll need to order or make yourself, but not all. And within those bread choices you will discover that there are a few forms of bread that are significantly lower in carbs than all their cousins and also have more fiber than most other breads. These types of bread products are not going to raise your blood sugar nearly as much as more normal bread. Allow me to introduce to you a couple of bread products that can become your good friends and allies in your quest to achieve normal blood sugar.

On the Store Shelves

There are no truly low-carb breads to be found in most stores. However, a few breads are at least "medium low." If I need to, I will certainly order foods or ingredients from online companies, but how much easier to buy it locally at a store five or ten minutes from my house! My go-to bread for sandwiches is Nature's Own Double Fiber Wheat bread. This bread has 11 grams of carbs per slice, but wait…4 of those carbs grams are fiber carbs. These will not raise blood sugar, which means that this bread has only 7 grams of blood sugar–raising carbs (or net carbs) per slice. This represents the lowest number of carbs in sliced bread that I have ever seen in a normal grocery store. And with only 7 grams of carbs, there are a tremendous number of things I can do with it and still keep my blood sugar levels in the normal range.

A 7-carb-gram slice of bread can easily be used to make "half sandwiches" (use one slice of bread—on the bottom, obviously), which will barely move your blood sugar. Pile some meat on that baby: a couple of slices of bologna, a generous heaping of turkey or ham or any kind of lunch meat. Add some cheese, a slice of tomato, some lettuce, and you have a nice little sandwich you can feel good about.

Some of the higher-carb breads have as many as 21 grams of carbs per slice. And if you eat sandwiches the traditional way (bread on top and bottom), the contrast becomes greater: 14 grams for the low-carb versus 42 grams for the high-carb! And don't think the difference between those amounts of carbs won't be reflected in your blood sugar levels and show up on your monitor! Find bread products that are low-carb that you enjoy, and stick with them, eat them, tell your friends about them, start a political campaign based on them…okay, maybe I'm getting a little carried away here! But you get the point.

Your diet and your health are in your hands. Nobody is going to force you to eat a super-sized box of McDonald's French fries. Whether you eat fries or a salad, whether you choose an avocado or some chips, whether you eat a couple of pickles or a huge cinnamon roll is up to you. Choose your foods wisely. Buy and bake breads that will not tax your pancreas and send your blood sugar and insulin levels through the roof, and you'll be a whole lot better for it.

The grocery store 7-net-gram bread does not compare with homemade low-carb bread that will probably have between 1 or 2 grams of net carbs per slice, but it's nice to know I can be lazy sometimes and just pull this bread out of my refrigerator or freezer, eat it, and have no concerns at all with blood sugar as long as I am being a good boy with whatever other foods I add to the meal.

Classic American Breakfast with Toast

One example of how I use Nature's Own Double Fiber Bread (7 net grams of carbs) without guilt is at breakfast. I will sometimes eat one slice of this bread toasted and smeared with sugar-free jelly. I add this to my eggs and bacon, which are going to possess almost no carbs at all. And with this one piece of bread adding only 7 grams of carbs, and the sugar-free jelly contributing perhaps 3 or 4 grams, I am staying under 20 grams, which I know is safe for me. Once in a while I will do a post-meal test after this, but in truth there is really no need. I know without a doubt that unless my body changes drastically, this meal will yield good results for me, breakfast after breakfast, and year after year. In the test below, you can see that my one-hour blood sugar "peak" is actually lower than my fasting blood sugar I had before I ate.

THREE EGGS, BACON, AND TOAST WITH SUGAR-FREE JELLY TEST	
	Eggs, Bacon, and Toast with Sugar-FreeJelly
Before Eating	97
After 1 Hour	87
Total Blood sugar Rise	-10 mg/dl

Summary: Who says diabetics can't have fun! Here is a thoroughly normal breakfast. I ate it, enjoyed it, and in the end my blood sugar went down rather than up after an hour. What gives? Apparently my pancreas was a bit tricked by the sweet sugar-free jelly and sent out a little more insulin than was absolutely necessary. Since there were so few carbs in my stomach for that insulin to deal with, my blood sugar was lower at the end than it was at the beginning. Had someone come in and seen me eating toast and jelly at breakfast, they surely would have thought I was a big hypocrite. But in truth I knew exactly what I was doing and how many carbs I was getting. I knew my body could handle those 10 grams of carbs—and it did!

Bagel Talk

Some forms of bread seem almost to defy nature in their tiny effect upon blood sugar. How in the world do they do this? Let's consider bagels. Bagels are an extremely thick bread, and as a result they normally have a lot of carbs. But not all! On the internet I was able to find a bagel that looks like a bagel, tastes like a bagel, and yet has only 16 grams of carbs—as opposed to the more normal 50 grams you find in most other bagels. But that's not all. Out of the 16 grams of carbs, 14 of those grams are listed as fiber, which leaves a scrawny 2 grams of net carbs to affect blood sugar in the entire bagel. Eating one of these bagels is almost like eating a small steak in its blood sugar–raising capacity. In other words, one bagel should have almost no effect upon your blood sugar. I know that's hard to believe, and I had to do a test on myself with this bagel just to see if it was really true.

The bagel is called the "Everything Bagel" and it is produced by the Great Low Carb Bread Company. There is one negative about these bagels and that is that you cannot find them in your local grocery store. You will have to order them off the internet. But they are so good and so effective at not raising blood sugar that they are worth it. Yes, the shipping cost is a bit painful, but if you order several bags at the same time and freeze most of them when they arrive, they are not terribly expensive. And in those times where you just feel like you're going to have to eat some bread that tastes like real bread, pull one of these babies out of your freezer, warm it up in the microwave, put some cream cheese on it, and ahhh… You have satiated your bread craving while your blood sugar goes nowhere.

Bagel Test

To demonstrate the power of fiber, I ran a blood sugar test comparing two very different bagels. First, I ate a Thomas Plain Bagel, which has 52 grams of carbs with only 2 grams of fiber, leaving 50 net grams to affect blood sugar. That's a lot of carbs! This bagel is traditionally what we think of when we talk bagels. It is big, it's thick, it's fat…and it tastes pretty good! But you are getting a lot of bread, a lot of carbs, and significant blood sugar rise.

To pit against this bagel I chose the Everything Bagel, produced by the Great Low Carb Bread Company. Like its high-carb cousin, it is fairly thick, it's big, it's beautiful, it tastes good (in fact, I like it better), and it has only 16 grams of carbs, 14 of which are fiber. This leaves only 2 grams of net carbs to affect your blood sugar.

When we put these two bagels side by side, we have 51 grams of sugar-raising carbs versus 2 grams of sugar-raising carbs. Do you suppose that might make a difference? I wasn't content just to read the amount of carbs and fiber and assume it was true. I wanted to see it for myself as it reads on my own little blood sugar monitor. From the numbers involved, I reckoned I should be able to eat three of the low-carb bagels and my blood sugar should still be significantly lower than only one of the high-carb bagels. And this is exactly what I did.

I decided to do the high-carb bagel first and get it over with. Before eating the Thomas Plain Bagel, my blood sugar read 108. I smeared it with cream cheese—after all, no bagel is complete without some cream cheese on it. But the cream cheese is quite low in carbs and would not affect the test much. I would be using cream cheese on the low-carb bagels as well.

Eating the high-carb bagel was pleasurable. It was tasty and made a nice little meal. I drank some water with it. During and after eating the bagel, I felt nothing going on in my body. This is part of the deceptiveness about diabetes and high blood sugar levels. You can usually feel it when your blood sugar drops significantly, but often you will feel absolutely nothing when it soars into outer space. From all my research and my previous blood sugar tests, I knew my blood sugar was rising, but I felt nothing unusual going on in my body. I felt fine. The only evidence I would have of what had been happening on the inside of me was the number that would show up on my monitor one hour after eating.

After that hour had elapsed, I pricked my finger with my lancet, held the blood drop up to test strip, and waited the required five seconds. I expected a number over the 140 limit I normally allow myself, and I was not wrong. The monitor read an ugly 189. All that doughy-but-lovely bread had done its job well. It had raised my blood sugar to a dangerous, organ-destroying, health-deteriorating level. Of course, I knew that my pancreas would go to work and get that blood sugar down in a few hours, and that I was not about to start eating this kind of food regularly, so I wasn't too fearful about ill-effects on me just for that one time. But if I ate foods like this regularly, I would be stupid not to expect some nasty effects showing up in my health.

It is interesting that in researching for this book, I had eaten a large salad with a similar number of carbs as this bagel due to its sweet dressing and crispy wheat strips, and my blood sugar had not risen nearly as much. Bread raises blood sugar much faster, much more thoroughly, much more efficiently, and just much more than almost any other food, save for sugar.

I waited several hours for my blood sugar to get back down to its base level, and finally it reached a much happier number of 93. Now it was time to eat the low-carb bagels. With 2 net grams of carbs per bagel, I would only be forced to deal with 6 net grams of carbs for all three bagels. I wasn't so much worried about a blood sugar rise as I was about how I could manage to eat all three bagels. One large bagel is pretty filling for me; two bagels would be a stretch. But I was going to have to force myself to eat three.

Normally eating three whopping bread products like these three bagels would send my blood sugar levels through the roof. I would expect to get close to a level of 300 mg/dl, which is quite danger-ous. But I was counting on all that fiber to save me and keep my blood sugar down in the normal range. Still, I was a little nervous as I munched on all that bread and forced that third bagel down.

Fully loaded with bagels, I waited for an hour to pass, eager to see exactly what my blood sugar monitor would reveal. Finally, it was time. With more than a little curiosity I pricked my finger and waited five seconds. The white on black number that appeared was a beautiful sight to behold. After eating three large bagels, my blood sugar had peaked at the one-hour mark at a scrawny 113!

HIGH-CARB VS. LOW-CARB BAGEL TEST		
	1 High-Carb Bagel	3 Low-Carb Bagels
Before Eating	108	93
After 30 Minutes	143	114
After 1 Hour	189	113
Total Blood sugar Rise	81 mg/dl	21 mg/dl

Summary: This is one of the most amazing and powerful blood sugar tests in this book. If ever there was proof of the power of fiber to restrain blood sugar rise, this is it. After eating three large low-carb bagels, my blood sugar never even approached 120! But after eating only one normal bagel, my blood sugar soared to 189—a dangerous level. The moral of the story is that bread can be dangerous for diabetics, but not all breads. There is a way of making bread, or buying it, that will be loaded with fiber and will not send your blood sugar into orbit.

As mentioned before, for the diabetic fiber has a double blessing because it is the only carb that does not affect blood sugar. The tragedy in all this is that any bread maker could make bread products filled with lots of fiber. But most of them just don't choose to do it. Ever since the discovery of white bread, bread producers have assumed that the finer the bread product, the better, and the coarser the bread, the less desirable. In truth, it is precisely the other way around.

If ever there was proof that low carb beats high carb all over the place, it's surely revealed in this bagel test. And to put icing on the proverbial (low-carb) cake, the low-carb Everything Bagels tasted just as good or better than the regular bagel. These bagels did not taste as if I was eating some kind of weird substitute bread. They tasted just like bagels are supposed to taste, but without the blood sugar rise. Wow! It doesn't get any better than that.

Bun Surgery

One of the simplest ways to make bread acceptable in your low-carb diet is to cut it in half. If you cut a piece of bread in half, what is left now has half the calories, half the sugar, and half the carbs. You may say, "So what?" But this is actually a powerful truth that can work on your behalf because many times we have our bread in pairs. A bun has two pieces, top and bottom. A sandwich has two pieces of bread, top and bottom. If we remove one of those pieces of bread, we have just cut our carbs in half! Now, with sandwiches and hamburgers, it makes no sense to remove the bottom part. All your in-between stuff would fall to the floor. But there is no reason in the world you cannot remove the top part.

Bun Surgery at Four Restaurants

To demonstrate the amazing effectiveness of this principle in reducing blood sugar levels, I went to four different restaurants to run some blood sugar tests: McDonald's, Whataburger, Burger King, and a restaurant at a nearby mall. From McDonald's I ate a McDouble hamburger, at Whataburger I had a "Breakfast on a Bun," at Burger King I ate a Whopper, and I ordered a panini from the mall restaurant. In each case I removed the top bun. With the Whopper I removed a little from the bottom bun as well because the bottom bun stuck out well past the edges of the hamburger patty. The panini had flatbread rather than a bun, so I tore off the top and side portion of the flatbread. I tested my blood sugar before and after each of the sandwiches.

BREAD-SLASHING TEST: HALF BUNS				
	McDouble	Breakfast on Bun	Whopper	Panini
Before Eating	93	106	93	97
After 1 Hour	123	112	137	136
Total Blood sugar Rise	30 mg/dl	6 mg/dl	44 mg/dl	39 mg/dl

Summary: Cutting my bread in half did not prevent blood sugar rise, but it definitely slowed it down. I feel tremendous satisfaction when I see one of those buns or pieces of bread on the table I did not eat. I don't just see it as bread—I see it for what it is effectively to me: sugar.

Full Buns This Time

After these tests I went back to the same restaurants and ate the same sandwiches, but this time I ate all the bread with no bread slashing. I was fuller after the meals, but the fullness wasn't very satisfying, knowing that by doubling the bread I had doubled the carbs and my blood sugar levels were almost certainly going to be significantly higher than before. As before I tested myself before the meal and one hour after finishing the meal. My results were just about what I thought they would be.

SANDWICHES TEST: FULL BUNS				
	McDouble	Breakfast on Bun	Whopper	Panini
Before Eating	102	94	94	98
After 1 Hour	149	162	162	147
Total Blood sugar Rise	47 mg/dl	68 mg/dl	68 mg/dl	49 mg/dl

Summary: By eating the full bun, my blood sugar did exactly what one might suppose it would. It rose significantly higher. With half the bread removed, my blood sugar was kept under my 140 limit. With all the bread, each of the foods raised my blood sugar over the 140 limit.

Eating the four sandwiches with half the bread, I averaged a 27-point rise. Eating them with all the bread, I averaged a 58-point rise. Interesting, isn't it, that when I cut the bread in half I cut my blood sugar rise in half as well. When I doubled the bread, I doubled the rise in my blood sugar. Looks to me like what was inside the sandwiches was inconsequential when it comes to blood sugar. But the bread that contained these ingredients was making all the difference in how high my blood sugar would rise.

Be a Saver!

The point of this is to be a carb-saver. Shave off as many carbs as you can, and you'll be better for it. If you were shopping and you heard of some items you really wanted to buy being offered at a 25-percent discount, you would become excited and head straight over to the discount section to see what was available. But if you heard that the things you really wanted were being offered at a 50-percent discount, you would think you had really hit the jackpot! And this is what is happening when you simply remove the top bun or piece of bread from your sandwich! You are getting a food that you enjoy at a 50-percent discount—on carbs!

Some people think it looks so uncool to be seen in a restaurant eating a sandwich without the top bun. So what? Does a drowning man get embarrassed when he is splashing around in the water and shouting, "Help, help!" at the top of his lungs? When your life is on the line, it is not time to worry about what others may think. And chances are most people could not care less whether you eat your sandwich with a full bun or half a bun. Some may object that without the top bun their fingers are going to get a little messy. Is that really a big deal? There is a thing called a napkin that works very well to clean off messy sandwiches after you have enjoyed your meal and slashed your carbs in half. So don't mind a few messy fingers. You've just done yourself a huge favor.

Muffins, Muffins

In the previous chapter I showed you how to make a super-quick "muffin in a mug." But sometimes I enjoy the old-fashioned muffins baked in a muffin pan. Muffins are an awesome breakfast food, and is there anybody on the entire planet who does not like them? A lifetime ago, when I was in my twenties, I used to eat two or three blueberry muffins every Thursday morning with eggs and bacon. It was such a great breakfast. I always looked forward to Thursday mornings. (I'm kind of a fanatic about routines.)

As with so many other foods, I slashed them from my diet when I started having blood sugar problems, but it wasn't long before I learned how to make a low-carb blueberry muffin from a low-carb cooking show, and I was able to enjoy them again. With some low-carb substitutions, you pay a high price in taste, but not with these babies. They tasted as good as the high-carb version, but instead of getting 30 to 40 grams of carbs per muffin, I was getting around 7 grams. Did my pancreas ever thank me? Well, no, because pancreases cannot talk, but if it could, I have no doubt it would have thanked me profusely!

Blueberry Muffin Test

I have been eating these same muffins for well over a decade now, and I enjoy them as much now as I did in the beginning. I decided to do a blood sugar test, pitting my low-carb muffins against some store-bought muffins that had more than 40 grams of carbs. I ate two low-carb muffins, and one and a half high-carb muffins. The results were exactly as I expected.

2 BLUEBERRY MUFFINS—LOW-CARB VS. NORMAL (HIGH-CARB) TEST		
	2 Low-Carb Muffins (14 Grams)	1.5 Normal Muffins (66 Grams)
Before Eating	105	103
After 1 Hour	107	183
Total Blood sugar Rise	2 mg/dl	80 mg/dl

Summary: No surprises here! Two low-carb muffins raised my blood sugar a total of 2 points! One and a half high-carb muffins brought about an 80-point rise! I think I'll stick with the low-carb ones. But the good news is that I actually enjoy the low-carb muffins more than the store-bought version. So not only do I save carbs and prevent huge blood sugar spikes, I enjoy my substitutes more anyway. God is good! For a low-carb blueberry muffin recipe, Google it, and you'll have your choice of dozens!

Benedicta's Response to High-Carb Muffins

On the high-carb blueberry muffin test my wife, Benedicta, offered to join me. Because she does not have insulin resistance, I bought her two even bigger high-carb muffins, possessing 55 net grams of carbs each. She ate both of these muffins, and her blood sugar rise could not have been more minimal.

BENEDICTA'S HIGH-CARB MUFFIN TEST	
	2 Blueberry Muffins (110 Net Grams Carbs)
Before Eating	97
After 1 Hour	99
Total Blood sugar Rise	2 mg/dl

Summary: I'm jealous! Benedicta's body is so efficient at processing carbs and sugars that she can ingest a whopping 110 grams of net carbs and her blood sugar jumps up a scrawny 2 points! If she didn't know better, she might easily do this test and conclude that blueberry muffins do not raise blood sugar. And to prove her point she could show that her blood sugar barely moved after eating two enormous blueberry muffins. But this proves nothing of the sort. Her test only reveals that she has a pancreas that works very well and little insulin resistance. This often fools a lot of people, and they criticize those of us who warn about fruit or rice or potatoes. It may not seem fair, but the truth is that some folks can eat high-carb foods (and have little blood sugar rise) while others cannot.

Some diabetics take a much simpler approach to bread. They simply do without it altogether—no bread, no bread substitutes, nothing that looks like bread, tastes like bread, smells like bread, or even attempts a poor imitation of bread will ever pass their lips. These folks would scoff at my idea of removing the top bun. They would argue, "Why not remove both top and bottom bun and cut your carbs still more?" This approach certainly works for them. It does not work for me. My philosophy about a diet that normalizes blood sugar and the sacrifices we must make is pretty simple: I will sacrifice what I need to sacrifice to attain close to normal blood sugar, but I will not sacrifice foods just to be a purist.

In this chapter I have attempted to show you that there are all kinds of substitutions or low-carb forms of bread that will enable you to enjoy bread the rest of your life without taxing your pancreas or driving your blood sugar level crazy. If you choose to go the way of the purist and never touch any form of bread for the rest of your life, more power to you. And if your diabetes has reached such a state that this is the only way you can get your numbers down to normal, then that is exactly what you should do. But if not, I hope you can get a few good ideas from some of the low-carb bread products and substitutes I have described.

The Other Side

If you do much reading and research concerning methodologies for curing, reversing, or simply escaping the ravages of diabetes, you will soon discover that two approaches seem to directly oppose each other. They are nearly polar opposites.

I am talking about the "whole-food, plant based, vegan/vegetarian approach" and the "low-carb, keto/Paleo, don't-worry-a-bit-about-the-fat" approach. People from both sides back their arguments with various studies and tests, and both freely give examples and case histories of individuals who were either cured or dramatically helped by going on their diet of choice. If you read the books and literature only from one side and watch the innumerable YouTube videos promoting that particular diet, you will be convinced that they must surely have the truth, the whole truth, and nothing but the truth. But when you start reading the articles and books by proponents of the other perspective, questions will come into your mind. *Perhaps the first group was wrong. I think maybe these guys have the truth on this whole thing.*

What are we to do?

Some may say, "I know the solution to this dilemma! I'll go with what the doctors and researchers say. I won't trust my own feelings or prejudices. After all, I'm not a doctor." Ah, but there lies the rub.

Doctors themselves don't agree. You can read impressive books with impressive stats, studies, and case histories by doctors who favor an all plant-based, low, low, low-fat, never-let-that-nasty-meat-touch-your-lips diet, and then find equally impressive books with just as many stats, studies, and personal testimonies by doctors who presumably studied much of the same things in medical school and yet promote low-carb, high-fat diets with eloquence and certainty. On YouTube you'll find the same thing. When it comes to a cure or reversal of diabetes, there are two camps with two nearly opposite views. They don't much like each other because the other side undercuts everything they believe, practice, and preach. Sometimes they get downright ugly with each other.

Bias

In order to understand the full story, we have to take a little detour and talk about the concept of bias. It would be nice to think that we are all so mature that we are entirely free from any prejudicial ideas and can easily accept the truth, even when it differs from our own background, history, or perspective. But the truth is, we all have bias on nearly everything. Show me a man or a woman who is entirely unbiased and wants nothing but the truth, no matter where that truth leads. I don't think there is such a person in the world.

When it comes to a cure for diabetes, the closest I've ever been to embracing the low-fat, plant-based diet was in that initial season when it was becoming apparent that I was heading down the same path as my mother. It appeared certain that I would become a full-fledged diabetic very soon. My blood sugar was bouncing up into the 200s after a high-carb meal and then diving down as low as 40 several hours after. At that time I didn't care a thing about being correct ideologically. I desperately wanted a cure, and it didn't matter from which camp it came. If someone had told me that eating dozens of frog's eyes every day would have driven diabetes far from my door, I would have scoured the local grocery stores looking for the frog-eye department!

My first attempt to help myself came when I read some information from an individual who promoted a vegetarian approach. He seemed to know what he was talking about and wrote with certainty, so I immediately cut the meat from my diet. If that was the price I had to pay to be rid of those terrible blood sugar fluctuations and living in daily fear that I would pass out, I would gladly swear off hamburgers, steaks, pork chops, and every other form of meat for the rest of my days. But when you eliminate most of the protein and much of the fat in your diet, you have to either replace it with something or else starve to death. And I did what so many people do when trying to be good and stay away from meat: I increased the carbohydrates in my diet. After all, as we have discussed, foods possess only three macronutrients: fat, protein, and carbohydrate. If you cut down on one of those, you will automatically adjust by increasing what is left. And in my case, this meant upping the carbs.

My blood sugar problems immediately increased about tenfold. My fluctuations before were nothing compared to what they became once I went to a high-carb diet. I got to the point where I had to eat about every three hours just to make sure I didn't pass out. And I constantly felt I was on the verge of losing consciousness. It was terrifying.

Thank God, after enduring about a month of this, I read some books that promoted a carbohydrate-restricted approach. What I was currently doing was surely not working. I had nothing to lose, so I cut my carbs significantly (but not totally), began to eat meat without guilt, and lo and behold, my blood sugar stabilized almost immediately. I felt normal once again, and my blood sugar levels stayed quietly within the normal range.

Low-Carb Equals Blood Sugar Stability

In the beginning of my struggle I was about as close to being unbiased as one can be, but once I found that I could achieve normal blood sugar by carbohydrate restriction, I developed some definite opinions about what diabetics and prediabetics need to do. And having kept diabetes away from my door for the last 17 years, I guess you could say that I'm not so unbiased these days. I'm not a doctor, I'm not a nutritionist, and I'm not an "expert" (except as pertains to my own blood sugar levels). But I know that carb restriction/reduction works. And it has not only worked for me, but for countless others. Type "low-carb diet" or "keto diet" in YouTube's search box and you will find more videos than you could watch in ten lifetimes. And they are increasing day by day, many of them posted by medical doctors.

I know, beyond a shadow of a doubt, that by adopting a low-carb diet, most type 2 diabetics can get their blood sugar levels down—fast! But what about the other side? Do vegans claim the same thing?

Well, almost. Of course, they cannot argue with the fact that when you significantly cut carbs, your blood sugar levels will decrease. Anybody with any sense and a blood sugar monitor knows that. But they argue that the low-carb approach is a Band-Aid, a crutch that, although it might work temporarily, will eventually lead to heart disease, sky-high cholesterol, poor nutrition, and an early death. They insist that their approach is the more natural approach. They insist that men were made to eat plants, not animals, and that when we eat plants and cut our dietary fat to almost nothing, especially animal fats, we will eventually find that our diabetes has disappeared. Many acknowledge that it may take some time, and that temporarily you may have elevated blood sugar, but they will tell you that if you just wait it out, sooner or later all that plant-based nutrition and vitamins will do their healing work, and you will see those numbers come down.

Are We Frugivores?

I have my own YouTube channel (type "beat diabetes pollock" in the YouTube search engine), and I am especially criticized when I suggest that fruit raises blood sugar levels. When I did the tests with Richard Clark, and he scored a 116 one hour after eating a big garden salad and a 199 an hour after eating a meal of fruit, some viewers didn't like that at all. I was told that if he would only go a week of eating nothing but fruit, those numbers would be fine. I wondered if they were really suggesting that the cure for diabetes is to go on an all-fruit diet, every day, every meal, nothing but fruit, fruit, and more fruit.

One man suggested that we humans are "frugivores" like monkeys and chimps. I find it strange that God gave us such sharp canine teeth just to tear into apples and oranges. Still, I'm not prepared to declare that everyone who claims healing from diabetes through a whole-food, plant-based diet is simply lying about it. Probably some have been helped by such a diet. My purpose in writing this book is not to tell anyone how to eat. I write this to share how I found victory in overcoming runaway blood sugar. If my experience can help you in your own quest, I thank God for it. Talk to your doctor, see what he or she thinks, and work out a plan for yourself.

There is no way these few and simple thoughts I will share in this chapter are going to settle the low-carb, high-fat versus the high-carb, vegan controversy. But for those who claim they have been healed by a vegan, eat-all-the-carbs-you-want diet, allow me to make the following observation: Any diet can be helpful in combatting diabetes if you end up losing weight as a result.

Suppose I convince you to try my "ice cream diet" (I'm using this as an illustration here—don't actually try this!). On this diet you will eat ice cream and only ice cream for the next three months. No meat, no fruit, no veggies—it's just ice cream, ice cream, and more ice cream morning, noon, and night. But I give you strict guidelines about how much you can eat. You are only allowed half a cup of ice cream at each meal, three times per day. With such a small amount of food, even though it is loaded with sugar, you will lose a lot of weight. Let's say that on this diet that you drop 25 pounds in three months. A loss of 25 pounds is significant, and in many cases such a loss will reduce your blood sugar levels from diabetic to nondiabetic. Many people are only diabetic when overweight, and if they can get to a normal weight, they will cease being diabetic. And any way they can get there, whether through an ice cream diet, an all-fruit diet, an all-meat diet, an all-sugary cereal diet, or any other diet that strictly limits calories and shreds weight, the results will be normal blood sugar.

But just because you dropped a lot of weight and ceased seeing diabetic numbers does not mean that your ice cream diet is the ideal solution for diabetes. Typically, anyone who gets serious about a new diet, almost any new diet, will see a loss in weight and will likely experience better blood sugar levels. But don't try to come preaching to me that I must immediately start eating bananas coated with peanut butter and steeped in pickle juice just because it helped you!

The Fruit-Lover's Two-Hour Post-Test Time Can Be Deceptive

One comment I have heard repeated in the comments section of my video posts about the potency of fruit to raise blood sugar is that I test myself too soon. They tell me that I must test myself two hours after eating, not one. They speak so confidently about this, it almost makes me feel they believe that when Moses came down from Mount Sinai, there was an eleventh commandment: "Thou shalt test two hours after eating." My response to these two-hour testers is pretty simple: "Says who?" Where is it written in stone that testing must be done two hours after eating? In most cases, that is exactly the wrong time to test.

Here's why (at least for me). When we eat meals, our blood sugar will typically begin to rise about 15 minutes after we eat. It will continue to rise for a time, and at some point, it will level off and begin to drop back down again (for type 2 diabetics) as our pancreas spits out enough insulin to deal with the blood sugars produced mostly from the carbohydrates in the meal. Ideally it will go down gradually but steadily, and at some point it will reach its base level. Then things stay pretty much the same until we eat another meal. When I test my blood sugar, I am attempting to discover the precise point when my blood sugar hits its peak. What I am trying to determine is just how far will a food or a particular meal drive my blood sugar.

Foods and meals with simple sugars and quick-dissolving carbs, like bread, candy, soda, potatoes, white rice, doughnuts, and so forth, will typically waste very little time in driving that blood sugar sky-high. Often within an hour my blood sugar can hit its peak and my monitor can read 200 or more (in cases where I deliberately eat a high-carb food or meal to prove a point—I would never do this otherwise). Then my blood sugar will start to decrease, and sometimes by two hours it is at a significantly lower level than it was at the one-hour mark. So if I did as the fruit promoters insist and waited to test until the two-hour mark, I would never fully grasp just how high that meal pushed my blood sugar. By the grace of God, my pancreas still works well, and it will dump out a lot of insulin to deal with those high-carb foods and meals. My blood sugar will not stay up high forever. It will peak and then begin to decrease.

What this means is that many of the eat-as-much-fruit-as-you-like folks are never getting a true picture of what fruit is doing to their blood sugar as long as they test only at two hours. Some might argue, "So what? As long as my blood sugar has returned to decent levels by two hours, I'm good. If it soared a bit at one hour, at least it didn't stay there very long. And my A1C scores confirm that I'm not a diabetic. So all that fruit is surely keeping me from diabetes. All is well!"

But all may not be so well. Jenny Ruhl writes, "No test doctors use for screening ever looks at how high our blood sugar is rising after we eat. So those post-meal highs may go on for years before they rise high enough to be detected. All the while, though, they are damaging our blood vessels and killing off our beta cells."[1] Of course, almost any food or meal will produce some blood sugar spike, but big spikes of 60 to 100 mg/dl are dangerous. I am not about to start testing myself two hours after meals when I know by innumerable tests on myself that my blood sugar typically peaks at about one hour for high-carb, quick-dissolving foods. Some foods, like pasta and beans, will peak later than that, so we need to consider the nature of our meals, along with our own body's tendencies.

A Mega-Fruit Test

Does testing two hours after eating tell the whole story? Benedicta and I put this to the test with foods we knew would spike our blood sugar.

Two-Hour Test

I heard from so many YouTube fruit-lovers that I must test myself at two hours that I decided to check this out. My wife joined me and represented "normal people." We both had a lunch of a large banana, an apple, and a mango. We would be ingesting between 100 and 110 grams of carbs, mostly natural sugar. In order to discover what was really happening to our blood sugar, we tested ourselves every 30 minutes up to 2 hours after finishing our fruit meal. At the end our results were pretty much what I expected they would be.

FRUIT MEAL: BANANA, APPLE, AND MANGO TEST		
	Dennis	Benedicta
Before Eating	114	86
After 30 Minutes	189	146
After 1 Hour	177	118
After 1.5 Hours	178	110
After 2 Hours	163	99
Total Blood sugar Rise	75 mg/dl	60 mg/dl

Summary: My wife and I both peaked around the 30-minute post-meal mark. After that our blood sugar began to decrease, responding to the insulin released by our pancreases. Had we listened to the fruit promoters, we would have waited to test at two hours and never would have an accurate picture of what the fruit was doing to our blood sugar. Even by two hours, however, my blood sugar was still way too high, at 163.

Even When Blood Sugar Numbers Are Decent, There Can Be a Problem

Let's say you feel you are healed on a vegan, high-fruit, high-carb diet. One thing no one can deny is that you are working your pancreas much harder than you would on a lower-carb diet. And what exactly is your pancreas doing? It is spewing out insulin. There is nothing inherently wrong or abnormal about a pancreas releasing insulin. It was made for just such a purpose. And if it ever stops doing that, you are in trouble. This is type 1 diabetes, and the only way to stay alive in such a case is to inject insulin.

Insulin, in proper levels, is natural and vitally necessary. But in cases where people combine insulin resistance with a high-carb diet (but still have a pancreas that functions well), their overtaxed pancreas is going to spit out three times, five times, or perhaps ten times as much insulin as would be normal and healthy. And when it comes to insulin, if a little is good, a lot is…terrible! Too much insulin floating around in your bloodstream is incredibly deleterious to your health. This condition is called hyperinsulinemia, and all by itself, even without high blood sugar, it can spell terrible physical maladies, especially heart disease. In addition, it makes it almost impossible to lose weight. Occasional high insulin levels are no big deal. But when it happens constantly, as in the case where someone with insulin resistance stubbornly insists on eating carbs, carbs, and more carbs, there is a big problem. Drs. Michael and Mary Dan Eades in their book titled *Protein Power* write:

> We know, as does every doctor, that the immediate effect of carbohydrate consumption is increased blood glucose, then an increased insulin level…As we studied the medical literature we found that *researchers the world over were finding elevated insulin levels associated with obesity, heart disease, high blood pressure, and diabetes*—the common diseases of modern man…These same researchers were beginning to believe (that what caused the problem in the first place was) the high-carbohydrate, low-fat diet.[2]

Oops!

In the '70s, prominent physicians, the United States government, and eventually nearly the whole world, erroneously concluded that the epidemic increases in heart disease, diabetes, and obesity were the result of too much fat in our diet. The food pyramid was born, and everybody and their mommas were preaching to us to get that fat out of our diet. The most popular boast on food packaging became the mantra "low fat." Millions dutifully cut back on meat, eggs, butter, and cheese, and gorged on chips, sugary cereal, and other "low-fat, heart-healthy" foods. What was the result? Heart disease, diabetes, and obesity went through the roof! We stuffed ourselves with carbs, our overworked pancreases wore out, and in the process we lived in a state of constant, excess insulin floating around in our bloodstreams. We got sicker and fatter and sicker and fatter. Thinking we were doing ourselves a favor eating bagels and doughnuts, and avoiding steaks and chicken, we were destroying ourselves as we submitted to the all-powerful, all-wise food pyramid that commanded us: "Thou shalt load up on the carbs and stay away from the fat!"

Drs. Michael and Mary Eades write:

> In the appropriate amount insulin keeps the metabolic system humming along smoothly with everything in balance; in great excess it becomes a rogue hormone ranging throughout the body, wreaking metabolic havoc, and leaving a trail of chaos and disease in its wake.[3]

Wow. That statement is so powerful and so important that little school children should be taught it right along with the Gettysburg Address. It might save millions from diabetes. At the heart of it is this simple thought: too much insulin can be very bad news! What does this have to do with the plant-based approach? It means this: even if by eating your vegan diet (especially if it is high carb) you are keeping your blood sugar levels near normal, you may very well be going through every day with elevated insulin, and that will eventually hurt you big-time.

Vegan Low-Carbers

Is it possible to be vegan or vegetarian and not provoke excessive insulin response? It is, but it is more difficult than it would be for a simple low-carber. You can eat substitute breads made of almond and coconut flour, you can eat lots of salads (mountains of salads), and plenty of nuts and seeds. It surely can be done, but I don't prefer to do it. Eating meat is both natural, pleasurable, and healthy for us. The Innuit (an

Eskimo people whose diet is nearly 100 percent meat) and the Masai (a tribe in East Africa who eat almost all meat and no carbs) both have thrived on high-meat diets for centuries and have virtually no diabetes and no heart disease. (It's a good thing that some well-meaning American didn't try to go to these people and teach them about the food pyramid.)

For those who feel they have achieved victory over diabetes through a vegan or vegetarian approach, I would offer the following evidence that should be present to declare that victory. First, your fasting blood sugar should not be much over 100 mg/dl. Yes, I know the official number that is supposed to mark diabetes is 126, but if your numbers are hitting around 115 or more, you are way too close. Second, you should have an A1C score in no higher than 5.9 or 6.0 if you're going to call yourself healed. And third, you should have your insulin levels checked and make sure that your "eat-all-the-carbs-I-like-as-long-as-they-come-from-plants" diet is not flooding your bloodstream with excess insulin and creating all sorts of problems of its own, even if your glucose levels seem pretty good. If these three markers all check out, you're doing well, and I would be the last person to tell you to change.

Goals for All

Whatever dietary and lifestyle plan you choose, there should be four major goals we all must share: 1) blood sugar levels close to normal levels, 2) we are getting plenty of nutrients by eating lots of nutrient-dense foods, 3) our insulin levels are not excessive, and 4) our BMI is in a healthy range.

Discuss these four points with a diabetes physician. If all these things are in order, you're doing great, whatever your dietary plan. Keep it up! (And why are you even reading this book, anyway?)

What We Have in Common

When you consider just how different the plant-based, whole-food, low-fat diet is from the low-carb, high-fat, enjoy-your-steaks diets, and the fact that both approaches claim numerous testimonies of people who have been helped by them, and claim victory over diabetes through them, it is enough to make you scratch your head in amazement. But when you take a closer look, you can find certain aspects that both plans share and that may make them more alike than they seem.

A good example of this is found in the book *The End of Diabetes* by Dr. Joel Fuhrman. Fuhrman's approach is essentially a modified vegan plan. He sharply criticizes meat and eggs and pushes a mostly plant-based diet, although he does allow for small, occasional portions of lean meat. He mocks the Atkins diet and criticizes any serious and deliberate restriction of dietary carbohydrates.[4] This places him at nearly the opposite end of the spectrum in comparing him with Dr. Richard Bernstein, who is my mentor and whose stress on limiting carbs has been such a revelation to me. And yet, like Dr. Bernstein, Fuhrman can produce large numbers of people who have been helped by his dietary and lifestyle plan. What gives here? Is he just plain lying?

I don't think so. When you carefully read his book and study the diet he recommends, you discover that he and Bernstein have more in common than at first glance. Let's consider some of their common emphases that may explain how two such widely divergent approaches to diabetes reversal can both prove effective.

Both Stress the Importance of Getting to the Appropriate Weight for One's Height

This simple but powerful thought, all by itself, could result in the cure of a huge percentage of diabetics and near diabetics. No, not every obese person is diabetic, and certainly there are some slim diabetics around, but carrying too many pounds increases your odds of diabetes, regardless of what you've been eating. Likewise, no matter which dietary plan you adopt, if you start losing weight and change from obese to normal, you may well end up one of the "testimonies" listed in the book of the doctor or nutritionist you follow.

Both View Sugar as the
Ultimate Enemy of Diabetics

Cutting out all candy, sweets, and sugary drinks is a must for anyone who is serious about getting control of their blood sugar, in both men's eyes. And, by the way, this is true for virtually every reasonable diet plan you can find anywhere. Try to find a dietary plan that suggests sugar is fine! You might hear this from the sugar industry, but that's about it. And, oh yes, the ADA (American Diabetes Association) strangely defends sugar, declaring:

> If eaten as a part of a healthy meal plan, or combined with exercise, sweets and desserts can be eaten by people with diabetes. There are no more "off-limits" to people with diabetes than there are to people without diabetes.[5]

Fuhrman responds, "This advice is flat-out wrong…As diabetics are given inadequate dietary advice, placed on medications that cause weight gain and push the failing pancreas to work harder and generally guided to mismanage their diabetes, the result will of course be more medication and the eventual need for insulin…This is simply drug-promoting doubletalk."[6] Dr. Bernstein could not have said it better. And as with weight reduction, any diabetes reversal plan that can get you to give up on sugar, sugary foods, sodas, fruit juices, sweet pastries, and the like can go a long way in significantly lowering your blood sugar levels.

Both Warn About Eating Starches

Bernstein views all starches as high carb, quick dissolving, and blood sugar spiking (which is exactly what they are). Fuhrman is not so quick to condemn all starches, but he does push people to lay off white bread, white potatoes, and white rice. He writes, "There are many vegan foods and vegan diets that would be unfavorable for diabetics, especially those that include lots of…finely ground grains and foods made from white flour and white potatoes."[7] He sounds a little like Bernstein, although Bernstein would say that white or brown, sweet or russet, all breads, potatoes, and rice have within them the ability to significantly raise blood sugar.

But Fuhrman goes a little further later in the book with an even stronger statement about starches:

> Typical vegan diets do not show the dramatic improvements in lipids, triglycerides, glucose, and even weight loss. One important design feature for better health and disease reversal is the reduction of high-starch vegetables and grains and the substitution of beans, nuts, and seeds instead…A high-starch, low-fat diet, regardless of whether or not the dieter is eating meat, can derail weight loss and lead to high triglycerides.[8]

Right on, Dr. Fuhrman!

Why Fuhrman's Diet Works

It turns out Joel Fuhrman, with his mostly vegan diet and his instinctive dislike for meat and eggs, isn't quite so far from Richard Bernstein and other low-carbers, whose basic concept for curing diabetes is to drastically reduce carbs, replacing them with protein and fat and lots of low-carb vegetables. When I first read some of Fuhrman's book, I thought, *How can this guy be getting results? With his nearly vegan diet, and the way he blasts low-carb diets, he is saying the exact opposite of Dr. Bernstein.* But when I examined his diet a little closer, I realized he and Bernstein weren't nearly so far apart. And yes, I can see why he is getting results with many people. Even though he refuses to put himself in the category of a low-carb dietician, by stressing the removal of sugar from our diets, and telling diabetics to beware of starchy foods and focus on beans, nuts, seeds, and green, leafy vegetables, the natural result would be that anyone who went from a normal standard American diet to his diet would certainly end up with far fewer carbs in their meals and should see significantly lower blood glucose levels. Fuhrman declares, "Bagels, white bread, pasta, pizza, and rolls are all staples of the American diet, and they are a large contributor to our epidemic of obesity, diabetes, heart disease, and cancer."[9] Bernstein and all the other low-carbers (including me) would have no argument with that. In fact, we would give him a hearty "Amen!"

Sadly, many vegan nutritionists and proponents are not nearly as savvy as Fuhrman. In their minds, anything that comes from the ground is fine. And some even go so far as to suggest that the solution for insulin resistance is more and more carbs. They see diabetes as a problem that can be fixed if we just keep on ingesting carbs until finally our body throws up the white flag and says, "If you can't beat them, join them!" The ADA recommends 45 to 60 grams of carbs per meal,[10] which is absolutely criminal and insane in the minds of doctors like Richard Bernstein.

What those who advocate a high-carb diet somehow miss is that what makes a diabetic a diabetic is an inability to process carbs and sugars the way normal people do. In many cases we got that way by stuffing our bodies with carbs and flooding our bloodstreams with insulin. And if we suppose that by doing more of the same, and more and more and more, we will somehow magically cure ourselves of diabetes, we are living in a fantasy world.

Adjustments

Life is filled with adjustments we must make. I wear glasses and have worn them for some time. I do this because I do not see well without them. I was not born with glasses on. You might say that they are "unnatural." But they are an adjustment I have to make to correct my imperfect vision. In an ideal world and in an ideal life, I would not need them. But life is not always ideal, and I do need them. Some people see perfectly and have no need of glasses. Their vision is 20-20. I do not judge them for not wearing glasses. They would be foolish to buy glasses when they don't need them. But neither should they judge me for wearing glasses. I *do* need them. And similarly, some people can eat huge baked potatoes, mountains of rice, and large amounts of the sweetest fruit every day. They can have pies and cake with ice cream for desserts, and still their metabolic system works beautifully, and they have no problem with high blood sugar levels. I do not judge them or insist that they must eat just as I do. But when they see me pass on the baked potatoes, or take tiny a little portion of rice, or say "no thanks" to dessert, or refuse that large banana, they should not judge me. I am doing what I have to do, and what is reasonable and right for me to do, given the fact that my body does not work today the way it did when I was ten years old. It is a very small price to pay for my health.

Thoughts About Sugar and Exercise

The rate of diabetes has increased dramatically in the US and many other parts of the world in the last 50 years. This is mostly bad news, but in one sense it is good news. The bad news is that multitudes suffer with this terrible disease in our generation, and the situation is far worse than in any time in our earth's history.

You may be thinking, *How can you possibly find any good news in this?* The one silver lining behind this terribly dark cloud is the fact that the rate of diabetes changes and does not remain static is clear proof that there must be something we can do about it. If the rate of diabetes remained exactly the same from generation to generation, from one culture to another, we would have to assume that diabetes is a completely genetic problem. If you are unlucky enough to have the wrong genes, tough luck! Take some pills or inject some insulin and hope that you can maybe last a little longer than some. "Why, oh why, did my parents give me the genes they did?"

But without question rates of diabetes can go up and down—and it's mostly going up these days. And this is true not just of diabetes, but of heart disease and high blood pressure as well. There are a cluster of diseases and physical maladies that in past generations in certain cultures have been nearly nonexistent. This hard and undeniable truth has caused some to refer to these diseases as "diseases of civilization" or sometimes "the diseases of affluence."

Meat Eaters

In Nina Teicholz's book *The Big Fat Surprise*, she writes much about societies that have included large amounts of fat in their diets and had little to no heart disease or diabetes. Nina says:

> George V. Mann, a doctor and professor of biochemistry... took a mobile laboratory to Kenya in the early 1960s in order to study the Masai people. Mann had heard that the Masai men ate nothing but meat, blood, and milk—a diet, like the Inuits', comprised of almost entirely animal fat—and that they considered fruits and vegetables fit to be eaten only by cows.
>
> Despite all of this, the blood pressure and weight of... these Masai and the Samburu peoples were about 50 percent lower than their American counterparts—and, most significantly, these numbers did not rise with age. Was it possible that we in the Western world were the anomaly, driving up our blood pressure and generally ruining our health by some aspect of our diet or modern way of life?[1]

If our current belief about animal fat is correct, then all the meat and dairy these tribesmen were eating would have caused an epidemic of heart disease in Kenya. However, Mann found exactly the opposite—he could identify almost no heart disease at all. He documented this by performing electrocardiograms on 400 of the men, among whom he found no evidence of a heart attack. Mann then performed autopsies on 50 Masai men and found only one case with "unequivocal" evidence of an infarction. Nor did the Masai suffer from other chronic diseases, such as cancer or diabetes.

In Africa and Asia, explorers, colonialists, and missionaries in the early twentieth century were repeatedly struck by the absence of degenerative disease among isolated populations they encountered. *The*

British Medical Journal routinely carried reports from colonial physicians who, though experienced in diagnosing cancer at home, could find very little of it in the African colonies overseas. So few cases could be identified that "some seem to assume that it does not exist," wrote George Prentice, a physician who worked in Southern Central Africa, in 1923.[2]

"Civilized" Diseases

In the British surgeon T.L. Cleave's book *Saccharine Disease: The Master Disease of Our Time*, he demonstrated through his study of numerous primitive cultures that they are almost entirely free of diabetes, heart disease, and hypertension—until a Western diet was introduced and adopted. He concluded that it normally takes about 20 years of eating refined carbohydrates and lots of sugar before the heart disease, high blood pressure, and diabetes begin appearing in a big way. But after that, their weaknesses in these areas rise to the level of all the "civilized" nations and they start dropping dead of heart attacks just the way Americans do and developing diabetes at similar rates.[3]

The evidence is becoming more and more compelling that it is sugar and megadoses of refined carbohydrates that are destroying our health, and not meat, fat, and dairy products, as we have been told since the 1970s. It is enlightening and rather depressing to research how it was that America and much of the world turned fat into a dietary bogeyman and convinced millions to cut their fat to a bare minimum while having no concerns or worries about the truckloads of sugar and carbohydrates they were consuming.

Yudkin vs. Keys

The "demonize-the-fat" and "ignore-the-sugar-and-carbs" story revolves largely around two different men who came to two very opposite conclusions in the mid-point of the twentieth century. The two men were British physiologist John Yudkin and American nutritionist Ancel Keys. Keys came to the conclusion that dietary fat leads to high cholesterol and high cholesterol leads to heart disease. Ergo, cut the fat out of your diet, particularly animal fat, and you will nearly eliminate heart disease. Yudkin, on the other hand, came to strongly believe that sugar was behind the cluster of "civilization diseases" that always surface when any culture or people begin to eat lots of refined carbohydrates and significant amounts of sugar. Yudkin recognized fat as something people have been eating for millennia, but refined sugar was a newcomer on the scene. Until the late 1800s, most people had little access to anything similar to table sugar. They might throw a few berries on their oatmeal or eat some fruit in season, but that was about it. There were no candy bars, no bowls for table sugar, no sodas, no cinnamon rolls—essentially no sugar as we know it today. Starting with this undeniable truth and then doing a great deal of research, Yudkin became increasingly convinced that much disease, and particularly heart disease, hypertension, and diabetes, would be nearly eradicated if sugar were cut out of the diet.

As the two men published their findings and wrote their articles, they became aware of each other. Yudkin allowed his findings and research to speak for itself, but Keys was more aggressive. He blasted Yudkin in his articles and essentially labeled him as crazy, fraudulent, or both. He mocked the staid British physiologist with flair and eventually was so successful in discrediting him that he created a climate where other researchers, nutritionists, and health writers became fearful of siding with Yudkin or daring to suggest that sugar and excessive, refined carbohydrates might possibly be far more dangerous than fats. Keys was not the researcher that Yudkin was, but he was far more skilled at PR. He won the fight hands down in the eyes of the public. Yudkin retired from his research but wrote a book that summed up all he had come to believe. It was titled *Pure, White, and Deadly*, and it thoroughly blasted sugar as being the premiere dietary villain primarily responsible for the degenerative diseases that afflict modern societies.

The American government got involved in the fray and sided with Ancel Keys. They published dietary guidelines for optimum health and recommended that we cut our fat to 10 percent of our diet or lower. They created the famous food pyramid we discussed earlier (later changed and then finally dropped), which showed carbohydrates as the food that should make up the majority of our diet in order to be healthy.

Just One Problem

It would have been perfect—if Keys was correct. But the overwhelming evidence indicates that he was wrong, dead wrong. Obesity went through the roof, and rates of diabetes skyrocketed. Heart disease was not stopped in its tracks; it rose significantly. Thinking we were doing ourselves a favor, we were in fact destroying our health. To put it in "Old McDonald" terminology, it was "A carb, carb here, and a sugar, sugar there. Here a carb, there a sugar, everywhere a sugar, sugar…" It was an absolute nightmare, a recipe for an epidemic of diabetes, which is precisely what we are facing today.

The reason I have not spent more time on sugar than I have in this book is because sugar is so incredibly detrimental to diabetics that it hardly seems necessary to belabor the point. Almost every diabetic knows they need to cut sugar out of their diets, but many do not recognize that starches can have nearly the same effects on blood sugar and resulting in high levels of insulin surging through the bloodstream and annihilating our health.

However here are a few quotes about sugar that state the case powerfully:

- Dr. David Samadi, chairman of urology and chief of robotic surgery at Lenox Hill Hospital: "Added sugar is one of the worst and most toxic ingredients in the Western diet. It can have harmful effects on our metabolism and contribute to the development of numerous serious health conditions and diseases."[4]

- Paul van der Velpen, head of Amsterdam's health service: "Sugar is the most dangerous drug of our time."[5]

- Alice Park, health and medicine writer for *Time* magazine: "Fat was the food villain these past few decades, but sugar is quickly muscling in to take its place. As rates of sugar-related disorders such as diabetes, obesity and heart disease climb, many experts believe that when Americans rid themselves of fat, they simply replaced it with sugar in all its forms."[6]

- Dr. Robert Lustig, anti-sugar writer and speaker who has become a YouTube superstar with his talk titled "Sugar, the Bitter Truth": "Every successful diet in history restricts sugar."[7]

The wonderful news is that by reversing the eating behavior that brought us to this diabetic precipice we can begin to back away and move toward good health once again. The old food pyramid is dead and buried; we are no longer under pressure to stuff ourselves with carbs and sugar. As we make the necessary changes, we will have the joy of watching our blood sugar numbers, in both our glucose monitors and our A1C scores, moving slowly (or sometimes speedily) back to normal levels.

It's More Than Just Your Sugar Bowl

To cut sugar out of your diet means more than simply throwing out the table sugar bowl that sits on our tables. We have to swear off those snacks and foods in which sugar is the main attraction: things like candy, cake, pie, sugar-filled snacks and breakfast cereals, sodas, nearly all "energy drinks," and the like. But we also have to recognize all sorts of foods with added sugar as dangerous. The list would be too long to name all our "added-sugar" foods, but the simplest way to guard ourselves against sugar-sweetened foods is to simply note the carbohydrate content on the nutritional information label. Often the sugar may not be called sugar. It may be listed as corn syrup, barley malt, dextrose, fructose sweetener, evaporated cane juice, cane sugar, cane crystals, corn syrup solids, and on and on. Rather than go over a long list of ingredients, simply go to the total carbs listed for a serving size (multiplying it to fit a real serving size) and see just how many carbs you are dealing with. Remember that a standard candy bar is around 35 grams of carbs. Anything approaching that is too much!

Must we give up on ever tasting anything sweet ever again for the rest of our days? Are we banished from sweetness and forced to live in dietary drabness and dullness forever and ever? No, we are not. There are two possible avenues of enjoying some sweet treats while still keeping blood sugar and insulin at normal levels. The first is through the judicious use of berries, especially strawberries. The strawberry is another one of God's gift to diabetics! (Yes, I know I have been a bit tough on fruit throughout this book, but strawberries and several other berries are exceptions.) An average-sized strawberry has a tiny little 1 gram of carbs! This means that you can have seven or eight strawberries (normal size), and you will only be eating 7 or 8 grams of carbs (I know…my math is dazzling to behold!).

Here is the second way to enjoy sweets: ordinary whipped cream is low in carbs. The brand I currently have in my fridge lists 1 gram of carbohydrate per 2 tablespoons. This means that I can have a nice bowl of strawberries with some whipped cream over them and only be taking in around 10 grams of carbs. But I don't stop there. I love to put the strawberries on a low-carb waffle. (I make these myself because I can't find them at the grocery store. Type "low-carb waffle" or "keto waffle" in the YouTube search box or in Google.) This waffle might add 4 more carb grams. And I know by testing my blood sugar an hour afterward that my body can easily handle this dessert. Life is good!

Other berries, such as blueberries or blackberries, are a bit higher in carbs, but they are still not bad, plus they contain fiber and their carbs convert to sugar significantly slower than candy. If you are determined to stay away from zero-calorie sweeteners, then berries and whipped cream are one of your best options for dietary sweetness. But if you are game for using some of those sweeteners, the possibilities are infinite.

Sugar Substitutes

Let's consider the issue of sugar substitutes, known by most as "artificial sweeteners." They are not all totally artificial. For example, Stevia is created from the leaves of a South American plant that has been used for hundreds of years in Brazil and Paraguay to sweeten tea. Some might argue that the stevia we buy has been "processed and refined," but of course that is exactly the case with the sugar people buy in five-pound bags. Do you suppose that table sugar grows as pure, white crystals? Splenda is made from real sugar. Erythritol occurs naturally in some fruit and fermented foods and is produced from glucose by fermentation with yeast.

Since the very first "artificial sweeteners" were available, the sugar industry has fought tooth and nail to suppress them and convince the world that they are death-dealing, health-destroying, and generally yucky. In addition to the sugar barons, many people who strive for a natural diet have had an instinctive aversion to them and have produced one argument after another to push us to ban them from our kitchens and our lives. It's almost humorous to watch them advance an argument against sugar substitutes and then drop that argument when it is disproven by research. Immediately they search frantically to come up with another argument, which they will preach with all their vigor until that argument is no longer relevant. In the last generation there has been study after study to try to discredit and forever banish artificial sweeteners, but to this day there has been no smoking gun.

Diet vs. Regular Soda

One of the things I have heard said is that artificial sweeteners "trick" your body into thinking that they are the real thing, and so your blood sugar goes up anyway, just as it would with real sugar. Now, that is an argument that even I, with no medical or scientific degree, could easily disprove, at least when it comes to my own body. Let's consider diet vs. "real" soda. If my body can be tricked by artificial sweeteners into raising my blood sugar, then I should see the same blood sugar rise with a diet soda as I do with a regular soda. I could easily find out if that holds true, as I did with the following two blood sugar tests.

REGULAR PEPSI (12 OUNCES, 41 GRAMS CARBS) TEST	
Before Drinking	102
30 Minutes After Drinking	152
1 Hour After Drinking	177
Total Blood sugar Rise	75 mg/dl

Summary: The sugar from soda hits your body fast! With no fiber or fat to slow it down, you get a lightning reaction to the 41 grams of sugar carbs, as my 75-point rise in blood sugar clearly demonstrated.

DIET PEPSI (12 OUNCES, 0 GRAMS CARBS) TEST	
Before Drinking	110
30 Minutes After Drinking	97
1 Hour After Drinking	98
Total Blood sugar Rise	-12 mg/dl

Summary: My pancreas may have been tricked a bit by the sweet taste of the diet soda after all, but not into raising my blood sugar. Instead, it released a little more insulin than it needed to. But with 0 grams of carbs to deal with, my blood sugar had nowhere to go but down. Comparing a 75-point rise to a 12-point decrease, clearly the diet soda was significantly easier on my blood sugar.

Some may argue that even though artificial sweeteners do not normally raise blood sugar, because they are artificial they are doing all kinds of hidden, untold, and unrecognized damage to our bodies. My first response would be to say, "Which artificial sweeteners?" They are quite different from one another, and it seems foolish to lump them all into the same category. And remember that plain old table sugar is artificial. It is not natural. To chew on a big piece of sugar cane would be natural, but to pour several cups of the white crystals into your cake mix or fudge concoction, or to produce a soda with 41 grams of the stuff in 12 ounces of carbonated water is entirely unnatural. What's more, sugar has been proven beyond dispute to raise blood sugar levels more than any other food (although white potatoes and white bread come mighty close).

John Yudkin, author of *Pure, White, and Deadly,* said this about sugar substitutes: "My own view is that it is highly unlikely that these do anybody any harm, whereas there is no doubt whatever that sugar can do a very great deal of harm."[8]

This is exactly what I have thought for a long time. The fact that researchers have been trying desperately for more than 50 years to find clear, unmistakable danger in artificial sweeteners and still they have almost no damning evidence to show for all their efforts says a lot.

Of course, if you are worried about it, just avoid all sweeteners, sugar and otherwise. Stay with strawberries and whipped cream, and small portions of melons. But don't allow the fear of sugar substitutes drive you to ingest lots of sugar every day, thinking you are doing yourself a favor by being "natural."

Exercise

In my previous books and my YouTube videos I do not say too much about exercise. It is not that I consider it unimportant. Everyone agrees that exercise promotes good health. My exercise machine of choice is the treadmill, with the elliptical trainer coming in second. Except on weeks when I am swamped with things to do, I normally try to exercise several times each week for 30 minutes at a time on the treadmill, although lately I've been doing a lot of old-fashioned walking.

When I first realized that I had serious blood sugar issues, I recalled a news piece I had seen years ago. It featured a Native American community whose men and women were coming down with diabetes in record numbers. Somehow several of these diabetics heard of the benefits of exercise in reversing diabetes and they began jogging. Their numbers improved dramatically, and more and more of these Native Americans began to jog. Remembering that story motivated me to get started with exercise, and the treadmill seemed the most convenient and surefire way for me to do it. In Texas we get blistering, hot summers and sometimes some pretty cold winter mornings, so having a treadmill in my house was one way I could always exercise in comfort, as well as privacy.

The exercise helped, but as I read and researched, and did one blood sugar test after another, comparing meals with meals and foods with foods, I realized that diet made a far bigger and more immediate difference in my blood sugar numbers than exercise. It didn't cause me to stop exercising—I have been doing it for many years—but I did come to the conclusion that exercise was not my number one weapon to beat diabetes. It could help, but it could never do for me what a dietary change, featuring significant carbohydrate restriction, could do.

Primacy of Diet

Research, case histories, and simply talking to former diabetics who got their blood sugars down to close to normal bear this out again and again. There is no question that exercise is good for you in many ways, but for the person wanting to bring those glucose levels down in a hurry, nothing succeeds like a radical dietary change from high-carb to low-carb. In the case of most type 2 diabetics it was primarily diet that caused the problem of high blood sugar and high-insulin levels, and it will need to be a transformed diet that brings healing and reversal of the diabetic condition. When you slash carbohydrate consumption, you slash blood sugar and insulin levels, and you may be surprised at just how quickly things turn around for the better.

For this reason, to focus most of your attention on developing an exercise program and spend hours each day walking, jogging, and lifting weights can be counterproductive. First, no matter how much you exercise, if you are eating doughnuts, bagels, and chocolate cake every day, you are not going to improve too much. And second, if you spend an inordinate amount of time out of your day exercising, there is an excellent chance you will never be able to maintain that regimen and will give up in frustration.

Verner Wheelock is a British scientist and a researcher who through a lifetime of nutrition and health research has concluded that the only hope for type 2 diabetics is to adopt a zero-sugar, low-carb, high-fat diet. Speaking of how sugar and carbohydrates overwhelm our metabolic system, producing insulin resistance and diabetes, he gives the following illustration:

> If I had a flood in my house…I would not spend day after
> day, week after week, and year after year buying buckets,
> mops, and towels. I would not be inventing different types
> of buckets and more expensive mops or drainage systems
> to ensure the water drained away quickly. I would find the
> source of the water and turn it off![9]

The point he is making is that, although various things such as exercise and taking certain medications may help a bit in reducing the flood of damage coming to us through high blood sugar and raging insulin levels, the smartest, surest, fastest, and most direct means to bring the ravaging effects of diabetes to a screeching halt is to stop it at its source—to slash our sugars and carbs so low that, regardless of what else we do or do not do, all indicators of diabetes will decrease. As no fire can maintain itself without fuel, no type 2 diabetic can maintain sky-high blood sugar levels without a diet rich in carbs and sugar.

Exercise and Weight Loss

Some may suppose that although exercise may not have a major effect on diabetes, at the very least it will help us lose weight, and our slimmer bodies will be more efficient in keeping blood sugar low. But the truth is that exercise is really a very poor way to lose weight. It can tone our muscles and improve our cardiovascular health, but its famous calorie-burning tendencies don't seem to be particularly effective. If you can burn off the calories from a doughnut by three hours of walking, why not simply skip the doughnut and buy yourself three hours to do other things?

Dr. Jason Fung has done a great deal of research on diabetes and is becoming, in my opinion, the premiere diabetes doctor for our current generation, just as Dr. Richard Bernstein has been to the previous one. Fung writes:

> In the end, here's the main problem. Type 2 diabetes is not
> a disease that is caused by lack of exercise. The underlying
> problem is excessive dietary glucose and fructose causing

hyperinsulinemia, not lack of exercise…Reversing type 2 diabetes depends upon treating the root cause of the disease, which is dietary in nature.

Having established that exercise is not your primary solution, let me back off a little and acknowledge that every diabetic should have an exercise program (under a doctor's care). It will help you—it just isn't your biggest weapon in the fight. If I were in the army and were going into a battle with a machine gun and a pistol, I would not throw away my pistol just because it isn't as powerful a weapon as my machine gun. It could come in handy, and in a battle, it pays to be armed with every weapon you can carry. So by all means exercise! Walk, jog, sweat, go to the gym, and do both aerobic and strength exercise. Muscle processes carbs much more efficiently than fat does, so toning your body should improve your metabolic efficiency.

But remember that the greatest of all exercises is to exercise your prerogative to say no. Say no to sugary desserts, say no to huge baked potatoes, say no to bagels, breakfast cereals, white rice, candy bars, sodas, sugar-laden fruit juices, peanut brittle, cookies, Texas toast, caramel apples, sugar-filled snacks, trips to the doughnut shop, apple pie with ice cream, apple pie without ice cream, and…well, you get the idea! Just say NO!

Bigotry, Ideologues, and Mr. Monitor

People who take diet and nutrition seriously tend to become ideologues. Their ideas and opinions harden to the point that they refuse to acknowledge there is any other correct view than the one they hold. If they are vegan, they mock the meat eaters and despise those who dare to suggest that any plant-based food could be even the slightest bit detrimental. If they favor a ketogenic diet, they cannot even imagine how stupid anyone could be to ever eat bread, potatoes, or fruit. And in the world of YouTube posts, these two sides battle it out ferociously, criticizing each other and making rude comments below any video post with which they disagree. I know. As I have mentioned, I have a YouTube channel (called "Beat Diabetes") and have to deal with constant criticism. I don't mind people disagreeing with me, as long as they do it respectfully. I don't hold a copyright on the truth, but there is a way to disagree with civility. Those are the kind of people I will respond to in the comments, and I don't mind getting into a little friendly debate with them.

There is one person who knows a great deal about blood sugar and diabetes, and yet has no bias or hardened ideology. You didn't think such a person existed? He does. His name is Mr. Blood Sugar Monitor. In my early days I read quite a few books and weighed various opinions. In time I came to recognize that carbohydrate-restriction was the surest and best dietary approach for me. It stabilized my blood sugar beautifully. But I didn't just come to this conclusion through reading books. Some of the books suggested this approach, but that was not what confirmed me as a low-carber. No, it was not a book at all—it was being introduced to someone who has become a great friend, Mr. Blood Sugar Monitor.

If there is one thing Mr. Monitor is not, it is a bigot. He doesn't care the least little bit whether you are black or white, African, Asian, Hispanic, or come from another planet. It makes no difference to him whether you are rich or poor, educated or can barely read or write, outgoing or introverted, highly intelligent or not so bright. He is not a vegan, nor is he a keto guy. He's not the least bit interested in your diet or how much you exercise or how many nutrition books you've read or YouTube videos you've watched. Mr. Blood Sugar Monitor cares about one thing and one thing only: the current level of sugar in your blood. How it got there, he doesn't know and doesn't care. That's for you to figure out. But he can tell you, fairly accurately, whether your blood sugar levels are good, bad, or ugly. You don't have to feed him or pet him or take him out to dinner. He is content to sit around in a drawer or on a shelf, waiting for the time you will pull him out and put him to good use.

Our Educator

And he can tell you a lot. He has given me a world-class education in blood sugar! He tells me what raises my blood sugar and what does not, when my blood sugar is at dangerous levels and when it is normal and all is well. And by using him over and over, hundreds and even thousands of times, he has given me an education in diabetes and blood sugar that, I am convinced, has saved me untold misery. As I mentioned earlier, my mother lost both her legs to diabetes, and the disease no doubt shortened her life. She had a blood sugar monitor but never did post-meal tests as I do. Consequently, she never really understood the full picture. "Cut back a bit on the sweets" was about as far as she took things. It was not enough. Nor is it enough for you. To merely "cut back a little on sweets" is about like throwing spoonfuls of water at a raging forest fire. You may think you are doing something, but in truth you are doing nothing. Diabetes is a ruthless disease, and our response must be equally ruthless.

Mr. Blood Sugar Monitor is not perfect. As we have seen earlier, blood sugar monitors still have a ways to go in getting to a high level of accuracy. But almost any blood sugar monitoring system can demonstrate incontrovertibly that a meal of ham and broccoli will raise your blood sugar far less than a meal of a baked potato and a banana. Those numbers won't just say it; they will shout it, and you would do well to listen. But you must learn to use Mr. Monitor properly, and this means going beyond the standard early-morning fasting blood sugar test. You must get started doing post-meal tests, testing your blood sugar one hour to an hour and a half after you finish your meals.

My Heroes

This is not to suggest we shouldn't continue to read and research. On the contrary, by reading great books on diabetes and watching YouTube videos we can not only learn a lot, but we can be inspired and motivated to stay in the fight and not give up. The goal is not to get blood sugar down to normal levels for a few months or a year, but for a lifetime. And this requires a little something called motivation. Motivation seems to be hard to come by for many, but in truth it really isn't that difficult to obtain. We tend to be motivated in areas where we pay the most attention. If you never read, never study, never watch talks given by diabetes educators, then of course you will find yourself lacking in motivation. So engage your mind in these things. Reading this book is a great start, but it is only a start.

And speaking of motivation through reading, allow me to introduce three of my heroes in the field of diabetes education who have all written some great books on blood sugar.

Richard Bernstein, MD

I have referenced Dr. Bernstein in each of the three books I have written. If you know his story you cannot help but be impressed with this man, who is a type 1 diabetic and keeps his blood sugar at near-perfect levels. He is now in his eighties and has helped thousands of diabetics. Here are three testimonies from people who commented after one of his posts:[10]

1. "My numbers are so good now after applying the advice contained in the book, my doctor has taken me off my liver and cholesterol medications...My A1C was 4.8 last week and my doctor says I'm cured. Of course, if I go back to eating the way I was my diabetes symptoms would return."

2. "Dr. B explains his way of controlling blood sugar with a low carbohydrate diet. It works. Despite being a type 1, I have an A1C of 4.8% as a type 1 and steady for the last 3 years and my blood sugars are between 70-110 a majority of the time."

3. "Nine years ago we began eating low carb. Within 3 months my husband was completely off insulin. Within 9 months he lost 80 pounds. Night sweats, gone. Apnea, gone. Neuropathy went from severe pain to a twinge now and then. Neurontin pain medication, gone. Diuretics, gone. He went from a man who could not walk 75 feet to a man who has now been in 2 5K races (walking) and who walks 2 miles 3 times a week at the local gym. His

doctor was astonished!!!! She said he was her "poster child for diabetics," and if she could get all of her patients to do what he did, she would be a happy doctor. But SHE didn't tell my husband what to do—Dr. Bernstein did!"

Bernstein is an author, a lecturer, and has a diabetes series on You-Tube called *Dr. Bernstein's Diabetes University*. He is well worth checking out.

As much as I admire this man, I have to admit that his books are not easy reads. He is highly intelligent and freely uses technical terms and concepts, and some of what he says, although no doubt true, is not exactly user-friendly. The other criticism I have is that Bernstein essentially strives for not just good blood sugar numbers, not just close-to-normal blood sugar numbers, but absolutely perfect numbers, the kind you might find in a 16-year-old with a perfect metabolism. This results in a diet so restricted in carbs that the sacrifices you must make are enormous. Whereas I am happy to have a fasting blood sugar under 100, he wants it in the low 80s. I'm feeling good if my A1C score is somewhere in the 5s; he insists it should be in the low to mid 4s, the level of someone with a perfect metabolism. I have learned a great deal from this man, but I've never felt the need to push myself quite as hard as he would if he were my doctor.

Jason Fung, MD

I have become acquainted with Dr. Fung in the last couple of years, and this doctor impresses me. His specialty is nephrology (dealing with the kidney), and any doctor who helps people with kidney issues is bound to come across a lot of diabetics. In his early days, Fung gave the standard advice and counsel to overweight diabetics (most diabetics are overweight, but not all), telling them to eat less, exercise more, and lose weight. He noticed that for many, as the weight came down, their diabetes lessened or sometimes disappeared.

But as Dr. Fung studied available research and the many studies that have been done with type 2 diabetics, he began to form what were at that time some rather unorthodox conclusions. Fung became convinced that a low-carbohydrate, high-fat diet was the one surefire means of helping men and women to both lose weight and quickly get their blood sugar levels down. The more he moved in this direction, the better results he saw with his patients. He soon became a true believer.

As he studied and worked with type 2 diabetics, he began to see that there was another factor that had to be conquered, in addition to high glucose blood levels, and that was high insulin levels. The more he studied and researched, the more he recognized that type 2 diabetes was all about high insulin. He became convinced that only the low-carb, high-fat diet could effectively deal with the high insulin levels that made diabetes an ever-increasing, destructive condition that led to heart disease, blindness, kidney failure, and could sometimes result in Alzheimer's and some cancers. In his mind, the biggest problem plaguing these diabetics was raging levels of insulin, and the only solution was a drastic and immediate restriction of carbohydrates, particularly all sugar and refined carbohydrates. As he urged his patients toward this diet, the results were fantastic. In his book *The Diabetes Code*, he gives numerous patient histories of men and women who have seen, not just good results, but amazing results.

But Dr. Fung found another piece of the diabetes-reversal puzzle when he discovered the power of "intermittent fasting." Through research and success with his own patients, he discovered that people with high levels of insulin resistance desperately need rest times, when the body is not constantly gorging on sugars and carbs and sending blood sugar and insulin levels through the roof. By encouraging type 2 diabetics to commit to a couple of times each week (or more) where they would not eat for anywhere from 16 hours (including sleep) to 36 hours, his patients obtained still better results.

Here are a couple quotes from Dr. Fung:

- "There were absolutely no tangible benefits to a long-term compliance with a low-fat diet…Despite forty years of research trying to link dietary fat, dietary cholesterol, and heart disease, not a single shred of evidence could be found."[11]

- "Sugar consumption rose steadily from 1977 to 2000, paralleled by rising obesity rates. Ten years later, type 2 diabetes followed doggedly, like a bratty little brother."[12]

- "The 1980 dietary guidelines spawned the infamous food pyramid in all its counterfactual glory. Without any scientific evidence, the formerly fattening carbohydrate was reborn as a healthy whole grain. The foods that formed the base of the pyramid—foods we were told to eat every single day—included breads, pastas, and potatoes. These were the precise foods we had previously avoided in order to stay thin. They are also the precise foods that provoke the greatest rise in blood glucose and insulin."[13]

Robert Lustig, MD

This man has become a YouTube sensation whose one-and-a-half-hour talk has over seven million views at the time of this writing. Lustig is a fine speaker, but he is not dynamic, and he uses all sorts of charts and graphs. It's hard to imagine how this man, standing still at a podium, never raising his voice, not telling hilarious jokes, and sometimes using words most of us have never heard of, has become so incredibly popular, especially when you consider his one main point: sugar is bad for you, even toxic. Robert Lustig has become America's premiere anti-sugar crusader and is quoted constantly by the low-carb crowd.

His research and his logic are impeccable, and it is difficult to see how anyone could argue with the essence of what he says. The truth is, he is confirming by study after study the thing we already knew: sugar is not a good thing, is incredibly detrimental to health, and is something anyone who takes their health seriously should avoid. He is essentially saying the exact same thing that John Yudkin declared in the 1970s in his book *Pure, White, and Deadly*. In those days when everyone feared and mocked dietary fat, few wanted to listen. Today they are listening, big-time. Find an extra hour and a half to view his YouTube video "Sugar, the Bitter Truth" and get his book *Fat Chance: Beating the Odds Against Sugar, Processed Food, Obesity, and Disease.* Here are a few quotes from this book:

- "Teens with type 2 diabetes used to be unheard of; now they are one third of all new diagnoses of diabetes."[14]
- "Keeping insulin low, eating lots of fiber, and avoiding added sugar. Now you've got something."[15]
- "The low-fat diet is what got us into this mess…First, a low-fat diet tastes like cardboard; the flavor is in the fat. So you up the carbs to compensate, increasing your insulin, and your weight."[16]

There are many other doctors, nutritionists, and various health advocates to which I could give honorable mention. The information is out there in abundance and it is readily available. With all the books you can order on Amazon and all the talks and videos you can watch on YouTube, there is no reason to live in ignorance. Not only will these resources inform you; they will also provide that magical, mysterious, and inexplicable factor we call motivation—without which all your knowledge means exactly nothing! So read books, watch videos, and get your motivation raised to a fever pitch. What you once considered a great sacrifice will come easy for you.

10

Final Thoughts

Throughout this book I have attempted to reveal to you some of the means by which it is possible for type 2 diabetics to achieve close to normal blood sugar. As I have read and researched, I have come to see that there are a couple of other considerations besides normal blood sugar that are also extremely important. In fact, they are so important that even if you get your blood sugar down into the normal range, but fail in these areas, you are headed for trouble. I've mentioned them in the book earlier, but I want to reiterate these things here at the end.

One factor is nutrition. Even if my blood sugar is in line, if I am not getting enough nutrition through lots of vegetables and occasional fruits (often half fruits) it is not enough. Low blood sugar is an intermediate goal, but good health is the ultimate goal, and that always means eating nutrient-dense foods. The good news is that the vegetable section of your grocers has all sorts of these foods that are jammed full of vitamins and nutrients and are also low in carbs.

The second additional goal is keeping my insulin levels down. Research is now piling up demonstrating that type 2 diabetics typically have two things working against them: high blood sugar *and* high insulin levels. This is why simply taking megadoses of insulin shots often does not reduce diabetic complications. Even though the added insulin may reduce your glucose levels, all the insulin you are producing, plus the additional insulin you are giving yourself, is making you a walking time bomb, saturated with insulin and ready to explode with a heart attack, a stroke, or all sorts of other physical issues. Dr. Jason Fung writes, "The major diseases of the twenty-first century—heart disease, cancer, diabetes—have all been related to metabolic syndrome and its common cause, the X factor. That X factor, as it turns out, is hyperinsulinemia."[1] It is much easier and cheaper to test for high blood sugar than for high insulin, but you can be sure that when your blood sugar is high, your insulin levels are high as well. The only exceptions to this would be type 1 diabetics who produce no insulin and type 2 diabetics whose pancreases are starting to fail and cannot produce the insulin they once did (which means they will soon become type 1 diabetics). When I first started having terrible blood sugar fluctuations, my fasting blood sugar and A1C scores were in the normal range, leading doctors to conclude there was nothing wrong with me. But my blood sugar was bouncing all over the place, which means my insulin levels were much too high. There was something seriously wrong, but it was not reflected in my fasting blood sugar levels or my A1C tests.

When blood sugar finally does reach beyond-normal levels, almost certainly insulin levels are quite high as well. This means we are on the receiving end of a one-two punch. Our bodies are being attacked two different ways, and if this goes on too long we will pay a high price for this. We are experiencing high glucose toxicity and high insulin toxicity. On the other hand, as long as your trusty blood sugar monitor shows you that your glucose levels are close to normal and are relatively stable throughout the day (especially your post-meal blood sugar peaks), all is probably well. This is why I test myself so often. Just as people use savings plans and retirement plans to prepare for a pleasant future in their old age, those 115s and 125s that show up on my monitor an hour after a meal are my way of planning for a nice, comfortable, healthy old age. I know there are no guarantees, but at least I am doing what I can, doing what I know I should do. The rest is in God's hands.

Doing What It Takes

In emergencies people do strange things. If your house was on fire, you might run out into the street in your underwear to escape the fire, something you would never do under normal conditions. You may be familiar with Aron Ralston's story. He was hiking alone and had his arm trapped under a boulder. He spent several days desperately trying to free himself. When he realized he would soon die, he did the unthinkable: He cut off his arm to free himself. He walked away and survived. (You can read about it in *Between a Rock and a Hard Place* or watch the movie, *127 Hours.*)

We humans have been programmed to survive, and when we perceive a serious threat, we will do about anything to get ourselves out of harm's way. The problem with diabetes is that it is such a slow and sneaky disease. We may have it 10 or 20 years before we notice various symptoms and start to get a little serious about it. But that is the one thing we must not do. We must take diabetes seriously before its destructive fingers claim various parts of our bodies and aspects of our health.

The number one evidence of diabetes is abnormally high blood sugar levels. In such a case we must take major steps to do something about that. One problem for some of you is that your diabetes is already at a point where your fasting blood sugar is far beyond normal. You may be waking up with your blood sugar at 150, 170, or even 200 or beyond. When you read about me focusing on blood sugar peaks at 140, you feel hopeless. Your blood sugar is already at 165 before you eat your first bite. There is no way for you to hope for a peak of 140!

And this is true—for now. But it does not have to stay that way. Fasting blood sugar is sort of like a report card on how you have been doing lately. When you've been gorging on sweets, sodas, mashed potatoes, and bagels, your blood sugar will reflect that. And even when you change and start cutting those carbs, it will remain elevated for a while. But eventually, like a reluctant child following Momma, it will start to drop as you restrict your carbs daily, weekly, and monthly. Fasting blood sugar is a follower; it is not a leader. As your normal meals give little reason for a major blood sugar rise, your morning fasting blood sugar will begin to come down. Richard Clark, whom I discussed in chapter 5, was walking around with blood sugar in the 400s. But after drastically cutting the carbs and going to a mostly vegetables and chicken diet, his fasting blood sugar retreated, and by the time I interviewed him a couple of years later, his fasting blood sugar was in the 90s. The level of your diabetes should dictate the level of your carbohydrate restriction. Because I caught my approaching diabetes before it ever truly became diabetes, I have never had to get too drastic with my diet. I just quietly and gradually started replacing high-carb meals with lower-carb meals, and my numbers came down beautifully. However, if I had not caught it so early, and my fasting blood sugar was 130 or more, knowing what I know now, I would take things to a whole different level.

Some diabetes experts recommend intermittent fasting, but there is another type of fasting that is a lot easier to manage: carb-fasting. I would set aside weeks where I would eat primarily meat, eggs, and low-carb vegetables—no fruit, no bread, no oatmeal, no cereal. Just meat, eggs, and low-carb veggies. After a week I might go back to a more normal low-carb diet with occasional bread, fruit, and so forth. After a week of that I would go back to a meat, eggs, and veggies week where I would essentially fast from all major sources of carbs. Blood sugar levels would go down, insulin levels would be cut drastically, and fasting blood sugar would sooner or later surrender and start coming down as well.

Like Aron Ralston, you do what it takes to survive…and thrive.

It Is a Great Time to Be Diabetic

I know it sounds weird to say that it is a great time to be a diabetic, but if you ever had to be diabetic, now is the best time in the history of our planet to be one. The research, the tools, the knowledge, and the testimonies of deliverance and reversal of diabetes are coming at us fast and furious. The fact that you can get a reasonably accurate blood sugar monitor and start monitoring yourself for $40 to $50 is fantastic. You don't have to take my word for anything, or this doctor or that doctor or this nutritionist or that nutritionist or the ADA or the CIA or any other organization. (Okay, so I got carried away! I don't think the CIA knows anything or cares much about diabetes.)

You can test yourself and find out what particular foods and meals are doing to your body and your blood sugar. You can watch YouTube videos for hours every day about diabetes and nutrition (including my YouTube channel, "Beat Diabetes"). You can order books from Amazon, and if you are reading the right books, you will probably end up knowing far more about diabetes than many experts, particularly those doctors whose knee-jerk reaction to diabetes is to put patients on a low-fat, high-carb diet and then prescribe insulin, insulin, and more insulin. You can sometimes even find A1C tests at pharmacies that you can do at home, but it would be good to have a diabetes doctor to discuss the results, particularly if your score is in the mid 6's or beyond.

And what is most exciting is that there are thousands of testimonies of people who have reversed their diabetes and are no longer classified as diabetics. Almost all type 2 diabetics have an excellent chance of achieving normal blood sugar levels, and the associated normal insulin levels as well. And amazingly, since metabolic syndrome diseases include much more than diabetes, by cutting your carbs and lowering your glucose and insulin levels, you will have gone a long way to prevent future strokes, heart attacks, Alzheimer's disease, and even some cancers. Birds of a feather flock together, and all these "diseases of civilization" tend to hover around two central components: high blood sugar and its evil twin, high insulin.

Before I adopted a low-carb diet, I had several conditions that bothered me for many years. Today they are all gone, vanished like a sugary popsicle on a hot sidewalk during a sunny, Texas afternoon:

- Frozen shoulders: I had the terrible experience of frozen shoulders that made me barely able to lift my arm. Don't ask me how this relates to high blood sugar. I just know that it's now a thing of the past.

- A spastic colon: This was a terrible condition. I never knew when it would hit me, forcing me to find a bathroom immediately. I had this for years, but when I went low-carb it simply vanished.

- Sinking spells: I had many, many times when I would feel I was about to pass out. It is a terrible thing to feel that you are losing control of your body and you could be on the ground in a moment. This was not caused by taking insulin. I have never taken insulin. I simply had an overactive pancreas that was going crazy as a result of my high-carb meals and foods. All of this disappeared when I stabilized my blood sugar with a low-carb diet.

- Arthritis: By my early 40's, I was showing signs of arthritis. At times it was painful just to shake hands. I was scared, wondering, *If I am this bad at 45, what will I be like at 60?* But by God's grace and a low-carb diet, I am better now at 65 than I was in my forties. The arthritis has been put on hold for the last couple of decades and shows no signs of returning.

All these things have vanished. Now in my mid-sixties, I am feeling much better than I did in my forties when I scarfed down breads, doughnuts, cereal, sugars, sodas, and desserts indiscriminately and with relish. When I first realized that carbohydrate restriction was helping me tremendously, I wanted to shout it from the housetops. I decided to write a book about my experience, titling it *Overcoming Runaway Blood Sugar*. I sent it to 40 Christian publishers, and it was universally rejected. Nobody wanted to take a chance with an unknown little guy like me. I was not a doctor, I was not a celebrity, and I had no degree in nutrition. I was just an ordinary guy with a story to tell. Finally, an editor from Harvest House Publishers came across a synopsis of the book and asked me to send her the whole thing.

I didn't know it, but she had serious blood sugar issues herself, and for this reason was eager to hear anything that might help her personally. She read the book, started applying the principles of low-carb eating, and found rapid relief from her symptoms of unstable blood sugar, shakiness, and leg pain. She became my biggest fan and promoter, and through her efforts my first book was published. I didn't know what to expect, but it amazed the publisher by going through printing after printing and selling more than 100,000 copies. By the time I wrote the second book, *60 Ways to Lower Your Blood Sugar*, they were eager to publish it. I held my breath, wondering if people would still be interested. They were! Up to this point it has sold a quarter of a million books and is still selling.

After that, I thought I had written all I could say or needed to say. But after reading a case of a man who compared the blood sugar rise he received from an oatmeal-and-toast breakfast with the rise he had with a Pepsi (both brought about a similar blood sugar rise), I thought this was one more story I could tell. Using myself as a human guinea pig, and incorporating a few other volunteer guinea pigs, including my wife, I began putting this book together. With the first two books, you had to simply take my word for what I was saying. But here we have test after test demonstrating what anyone with any sense who studies diabetes should know: high carb equals high blood sugar; low carb equals lower blood sugar. It is not profound, it is not particularly deep, but it is powerful, and it is true!

This book is the result of uncountable blood sugar tests. I am fully aware that these tests do not qualify as a scientific study. The monitors I used weren't terribly expensive, and you certainly have to allow for a margin of error. But the main point is overwhelmingly clear and cannot be reasonably opposed. More importantly, you can do these tests on yourself if you don't trust my evidence.

Take advantage of this wonderful time in which we live. To paraphrase Mr. Dickens, "It is the best of times and the worst of times." Our world has a lot of problems, but at least in the area of type 2 diabetes, the answers are readily available. The studies and the research are increasing at such a rate that the day will come when the answers will no longer be up for debate. But until then you'll have to do a little research and make a few judgments on your own. But that's okay. You can do it. Ask God's help. We have it on good authority that He gives generously to those who ask Him for wisdom (James 1:5).

Just a Starter

I fully realize the limitations of this book. I am a simple guy, a Bible teacher, who faced the awful prospect of diabetes and dodged a bullet 17 years ago. There are all kinds of doctors and researchers who are smarter than I am, more educated than I am, and have more degrees than I have. Let this book be your "starter," not your diabetes manual.

But there is one subject upon which I am uniquely qualified to expound: my own body and its blood sugar response to foods of all kinds. I suppose by this time I have performed thousands of blood sugar tests on myself. I have learned a lot through this process, and what I have learned has led me on the path of a carbohydrate-restricted diet, with the result of stable blood sugar and nondiabetic blood sugar levels, as reflected in fasting blood sugar tests and in my A1C tests.

The other day when talking with someone who asked me if I was diabetic, I responded, "No, but if I ate like everybody else does, I surely would be!" I truly believe this, and I thank God for intervening in my life early on, before things got entirely out of hand.

I have not written this to make converts, to make little "Dennises" all over the world. If your path leads you to a different dietary plan, and results in normal blood sugar and reasonable insulin levels, I am happy for you. My goal is to inspire normal, everyday folks who probably would not benefit from a book filled with a lot of technical terms and words they never heard of. My main message is the simple thought that there really is hope for you to escape type 2 diabetes and live the rest of your days free from it. I recently interviewed a policeman who went from an A1C of 10.0 to 5.8 in the space of three months through carbohydrate restriction. Another interview I posted on YouTube featured a man who went from an A1C of 14.0 to 5.0 by cutting his carbs. You can do it too! Work with your doctor, read, research, watch videos, test, practice a little self-denial, pray—and test and pray some more. And by all means become close friends with your blood sugar monitor. He has a lot to teach you.

Bonus Material

The following pages are here for you in case you would like to try your own blood sugar tests with the book at hand. Once you are familiar with them, you can start your own journal or other method of keeping a record of your tests and results. They will change your life!

Food Choices

Breakfast: _____

_____

_____

_____

_____

_____

_____

_____

Lunch: _____

_____

_____

_____

_____

_____

_____

Dinner: _____

_____

_____

_____

_____

_____

_____

Blood Sugar Test Results and Summary

Before	
30 Minutes After	
1 Hour After	
Total Blood Sugar Rise	
Summary:	

Before	
30 Minutes After	
1 Hour After	
Total Blood Sugar Rise	
Summary:	

Before	
30 Minutes After	
1 Hour After	
Total Blood Sugar Rise	
Summary:	

Food Choices

Breakfast: _____

_____

_____

_____

_____

_____

_____

Lunch: _____

_____

_____

_____

_____

_____

_____

Dinner: _____

_____

_____

_____

_____

_____

_____

Blood Sugar Test Results and Summary

Before	
30 Minutes After	
1 Hour After	
Total Blood Sugar Rise	
Summary:	

Before	
30 Minutes After	
1 Hour After	
Total Blood Sugar Rise	
Summary:	

Before	
30 Minutes After	
1 Hour After	
Total Blood Sugar Rise	
Summary:	

Food Choices

Breakfast: _____

_____

_____

_____

_____

_____

_____

Lunch: _____

_____

_____

_____

_____

_____

_____

Dinner: _____

_____

_____

_____

_____

_____

_____

Blood Sugar Test Results and Summary

Before	
30 Minutes After	
1 Hour After	
Total Blood Sugar Rise	
Summary:	

Before	
30 Minutes After	
1 Hour After	
Total Blood Sugar Rise	
Summary:	

Before	
30 Minutes After	
1 Hour After	
Total Blood Sugar Rise	
Summary:	

Food Choices

Breakfast: _____

_____

_____

_____

_____

_____

_____

_____

Lunch: _____

_____

_____

_____

_____

_____

_____

_____

Dinner: _____

_____

_____

_____

_____

_____

_____

_____

Blood Sugar Test Results and Summary

Before	
30 Minutes After	
1 Hour After	
Total Blood Sugar Rise	
Summary:	

Before	
30 Minutes After	
1 Hour After	
Total Blood Sugar Rise	
Summary:	

Before	
30 Minutes After	
1 Hour After	
Total Blood Sugar Rise	
Summary:	

Food Choices

Breakfast: _____

_____

_____

_____

_____

_____

_____

_____

Lunch: _____

_____

_____

_____

_____

_____

_____

_____

Dinner: _____

_____

_____

_____

_____

_____

_____

_____

Blood Sugar Test Results and Summary

Before	
30 Minutes After	
1 Hour After	
Total Blood Sugar Rise	
Summary:	

Before	
30 Minutes After	
1 Hour After	
Total Blood Sugar Rise	
Summary:	

Before	
30 Minutes After	
1 Hour After	
Total Blood Sugar Rise	
Summary:	

Food Choices

Breakfast: _____

_____

_____

_____

_____

_____

_____

_____

Lunch: _____

_____

_____

_____

_____

_____

_____

_____

Dinner: _____

_____

_____

_____

_____

_____

_____

_____

Blood Sugar Test Results and Summary

Before	
30 Minutes After	
1 Hour After	
Total Blood Sugar Rise	
Summary:	

Before	
30 Minutes After	
1 Hour After	
Total Blood Sugar Rise	
Summary:	

Before	
30 Minutes After	
1 Hour After	
Total Blood Sugar Rise	
Summary:	

Notes

Chapter 1: My Story

1. Semanticscholar.org, American Association of Clinical Endocrinologists Medical Guidelines for Clinical Practice for the Management of Diabetes Mellitus, Endocrine Practice Vol 13 (Suppl 1) May/June 2007, https://pdfs.semanticscholar.org/98e8/e80aa77d1a42fec21d3eb392dece1baeefa 6.pdf.

2. Sarah Hallberg, "Reversing Type 2 diabetes starts with ignoring the guidelines," YouTube.com, May 4, 2015, https://www.youtube.com/watch?v=da1vvigy5tQ&t=756s.

3. Robert Atkins, *Dr. Atkins' New Diet Revolution* (Lanham, MD; Government Institutes, 2002), 190.

Chapter 2: Let's Talk About Blood Sugar Testing

1. Dr. Richard Bernstein, *Dr. Bernstein's Diabetes University*, "Introduction," YouTube, December 9, 2014, https://www.youtube.com/watch?v=WFNGdKSXx64&t=7s.

2. Jenny Ruhl, *Blood Sugar 101* (Turners Falls, MA: Technion Books, 2008), 82.

3. Ibid.

Chapter 3: Check Those Labels!

1. M. Ward, "Thoughts about Food Politics," November 3, 2008, http://mwardfoodpolitics .blogspot.com/2008/11/chapter-11-making-health-claims-legal_30.html.

2. Dr. Richard Bernstein, *Dr. Bernstein's Diabetes University*, "Should Diabetics Eat Fruit?" YouTube, September 26, 2015, https://www.youtube.com/watch?v=2_odM7TZwtM.

Chapter 4: Breakfast: Getting a Good Start

1. Google search, https://www.google.com/search?q=definition+of+pragmatic&rlz=1C1CHWA_ enUS648US649&oq=definition+of+pragmatic&aqs=chrome..69i57j0l5.5838j1j8&sourceid= chrome&ie=UTF-8.

2. Gary Taubes, *Why We Get Fat* (New York, NY; Anchor Books, 2010), 9-10.

3. Dr. Jason Fung, *The Diabetes Code* (Vancouver, Canada: Greystone Books, 2018), 8-10.

4. Craig Clarke, "What Is the Best Triglyceride Lowering Diet?" Ruled.me, https://www.ruled.me/ best-triglyceride-lowering-diet/.

5. Susan Scutti, "An egg a day might reduce your risk of heart disease, study says," CNN.com, May 21, 2018, https://www.cnn.com/2018/05/21/health/eggs-heart-disease-study/index.html.

Chapter 6: The Big Four Starches

1. Franziska Spritzler, *Carbohydrate Restriction*, "The Key to Achieving Optimal Blood Sugar," You Tube.com, October 10, 2014, https://www.youtube.com/watch?v=op6WBOsJiuw&t=257s.

2. Jenny Ruhl, *Blood Sugar 101* (Turners Falls, MA: Technion Books, 2008), 69.

3. Laura Dolson, "Understanding Complex Carbohydrates," verywellfit.com, September 19, 2018, https://www.verywellfit.com/what-you-need-to-know-about-complex-carbohydrates-2242228.

4. Kris Gunnars, "Is Bread Bad for Your Health?" healthline.com, February 6, 2013, https://www.healthline.com/nutrition/why-is-bread-bad-for-you.

5. Barbie Cervoni, "Is Dreamfields Pasta Really Low-Carb?" verywellhealth.com, June 13, 2018, https://www.verywellhealth.com/dreamfields-pasta-a-hoax-1087507.

6. Laura Dolson, "Why Do Potatoes Have a Higher Glycemic Index Than Sugar?" verywellfit.com, June 28, 2018, https://www.verywellfit.com/why-do-potatoes-raise-blood-glucose-more-than-sugar-2242317.

Chapter 7: More About Bread

1. "15 Ways High Blood Sugar Affects Your Body," Health.com, https://www.health.com/type-2-diabetes/high-blood-sugar-symptoms?slide=372017#372017.

2. American Diabetes Association, "What type of damage does high blood glucose do to my body?" sharecare.com, https://www.sharecare.com/health/hyperglycemia/type-of-damage-high-blood-glucose-does-to-body.

3. National Kidney Foundation, "Diabetes and Your Eyes, Heart, Nerves, Feet, and Kidneys," kidney.org, https://www.kidney.org/atoz/content/Diabetes-and-Your-Eyes-Heart-Nerves-Feet-and-Kidneys.

4. Dr. Richard Bernstein, "The Basic Food Groups: Carbohydrate," diabetes-book.com, http://www.diabetes-book.com/carbohydrate/.

Chapter 8: The Other Side

1. Jenny Ruhl, *Your Diabetes Questions Answered* (Turners Falls, MA: Technion Books, 2017), 45.

2. Drs. Michael and Mary Eades, *Protein Power* (New York, NY: Bantam Books, 1996), xiv.

3. Ibid., 24.

4. Dr. Joel Fuhrman, *The End of Diabetes* (New York, NY: HarperOne, 2013).

5. Ibid., 36.

6. Ibid., 37.

7. Ibid., 114.

8. Ibid., 115.

9. Ibid., 93.

10. " All About Carbohydrate Counting," professionaldiabetes.org, https://professional.diabetes.org/sites/professional.diabetes.org/files/media/All_About_Carbohydrate_Counting.pdf.

Chapter 9: Thoughts About Sugar and Exercise

1. Nina Teicholz, *The Big Fat Surprise* (New York, NY: Simon & Schuster Paperbacks, 2015), 11-12.

2. Robert Atkins, *Dr. Atkins' New Diet Revolution* (New York, NY: Avon Books, 1992), 359.

3. Ibid., 314.

4. Dr. David Samadi, "Sugar Is Not Only a Drug but a Poison Too," Huffpost.com, January 6, 2016, https://www.huffpost.com/entry/sugar-is-not-only-a-drug-but-a-poison-too_b_8918630.

5. Emma Innes, "Sugar Is 'the Most Dangerous Drug of Our Time,'" Daily Mail.com, September 18, 2013, https://www.dailymail.co.uk/health/article-2424396/Sugar-dangerous-drug-time-come-smoking-style-health-warnings-says-Dutch-health-chief.html.

6. Alice Park, "Sugar Is Definitely Toxic, a New Study Says," Time, October 27, 2015, http://time.com/4087775/sugar-is-definitely-toxic-a-new-study-says/.

7. Dr. Robert Lustig, *Fat Chance* (New York, NY: Plume, 2013), 117.

8. John Yudkin, *Pure, White, and Deadly* (New York, NY: Penguin Books, 1972), 185.

9. Dr. Jason Fung, *The Diabetes Code* (Vancouver, Canada: Greystone Books, 2018), 173.

10. Amazon reviews for Dr. Richard Bernstein's book *Dr. Bernstein's Diabetes Solution: The Complete Guide to Achieving Normal Blood Sugar*s, amazon.com, https://www.amazon.com/Dr-Bernsteins-Diabetes-Solution-Achieving/product-reviews/0316182699.

11. Dr. Jason Fung, *The Diabetes Code* (Vancouver, Canada: Greystone Books, 2018), 154.

12. Ibid., 95.

13. Ibid., 9.

14. Dr. Robert Lustig, *Fat Chance* (New York, NY: Plume, 2013), 4.

15. Ibid., 131.

16. Ibid., 185.

Chapter 10: Final Thoughts

1. Dr. Jason Fung, *The Diabetes Code* (Vancouver, Canada: Greystone Books, 2018), 108.

About Dennis Pollock and Spirit of Grace Ministries

Dennis Pollock is the founder and president of Spirit of Grace Ministries. His primary work in this ministry is to write and record devotional biblical articles and to hold mission conferences and evangelistic outreaches in Africa. However, he also considers the sharing of his testimony of deliverance from diabetes an important aspect of the ministry. You can learn more about his ministry by visiting the website: **www.spiritofgrace.org**.

Many of the tests and concepts you read about in this book may be found on Dennis's YouTube channel, titled "Beat Diabetes." To find Dennis's many videos about blood sugar, go to YouTube and type "Beat Diabetes Pollock" in the YouTube search box. By subscribing to the channel, you will be notified as new videos are posted.

Dennis would love to hear from you! Feel free to email him and share your journey with blood sugar issues or your journey with the Lord Jesus. Dennis has written over 400 devotional articles on all sorts of biblical topics. You can find these by going Dennis's website and then clicking on the picture of the Bible in front of a fireplace. These articles have also been recorded as mp3 files and may be downloaded from our devo catalogue page. You can also see abbreviated "video devos" on his ministry YouTube channel. Go to the YouTube search engine and type "Dennis Pollock" in the search box.

Spirit of Grace Ministries
PO Box 2068
McKinney, TX 75070
Website: www.spiritofgrace.org
Email: grace@spiritofgrace.org

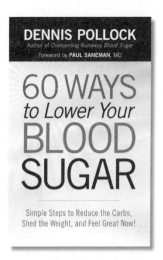

DENNIS POLLOCK
Author of *Overcoming Runaway Blood Sugar*
Foreword by **PAUL SANEMAN**, MD

60 WAYS
to Lower Your
BLOOD
SUGAR

Simple Steps to Reduce the Carbs,
Shed the Weight, and Feel Great Now!

Lose Weight, Boost Your Energy, and Feel Better—for Life!

Could it be this simple? Cut down carbs, add some exercise—and you'll reduce your blood sugar, lose weight, and maybe save your life?

The seriously out-of-whack American diet has led to rampant obesity and a myriad of prediabetic and diabetic problems for tens of millions. Step off the high-carb, bad-health train as Dennis Pollock, author of *Overcoming Runaway Blood Sugar*, gives you 60 practical tips, ideas, and actions you can take to...

- reduce your carb intake without resorting to a dreary diet of unvarying and uninteresting meals
- start exercising in ways that fit into real life
- stay motivated as you regain your health and see long-term benefits

If you're ready to stop paying the high cost of high blood sugar, here's a realistic, one-change-at-a-time plan to feel great, restore your energy, and live a better and longer life.